PROSTATE

"IF YOU SEEK GUIDANCE AND INFORMATION CONCERNING THE PROBLEMS THAT FACE THE PROSTATE SUFFERER, THEN YOU HAVE FOUND A MARVELOUS SOURCE BOOK.

"I RECOMMEND *THE PROSTATE PROBLEM* HIGHLY, NOT AS A SUBSTITUTE FOR GOOD MEDICAL ADVICE, BUT AS A TOOL FOR MAKING BETTER, MORE INFORMED MEDICAL CHOICES."

—*Dr. Israel Barken,*
from his Foreword to
THE PROSTATE PROBLEM

THE PROSTATE PROBLEM
Get the facts . . . they could save your life!

THE PROSTATE PROBLEM

THE GUIDE TO WHAT EVERY MAN OVER 40 NEEDS TO KNOW AND WHY!

CHET CUNNINGHAM

With a Foreword by
Dr. Israel Barken, M.D. F.A.C.S. Urology, Beard Certified

PINNACLE BOOKS
WINDSOR PUBLISHING CORP.

PINNACLE BOOKS are published by

Windsor Publishing Corp.
475 Park Avenue South
New York, NY 10016

First Pinnacle Books Printing: August, 1993

Printed in the United States of America

Dedicated to all of those men who ignored the symptoms, refused to believe the diagnosis, and failed to act quickly enough to save their own lives. May the rest of us learn from their experiences. May we all survive "the prostate years" and not die until we're 95 doing exactly what we want to do!

Contents

Foreword

As residents learning to treat patients in the clinics of Barnes Hospital, St. Louis, we would tremble when we did grand rounds and the Chief of Urology demanded, "How should we treat this patient?" The answer had to be correct, sharp, and decisive.

After years of clinical practice and meeting thousands of men and women looking to me for an answer, I have learned to ask, "What does *this patient* want to do?"

One of the skills of a physician is getting to know a patient—finding out what he wants, which options he can choose from, which treatments he can tolerate physically and psychologically, what his belief systems are, and how he can use his keen powers of mind and body in the process of getting well.

Perhaps you bought this book to find out about some of the exciting technology that has revolutionized the practice of urology. We now have sound waves that can break up stones, we have ultrasound to give us eyes into deep cavities of the body, we perform surgery through high-powered microscopes and miniaturized cameras, we have harnessed the power of the laser to melt away tissue, and we have refined cryosurgery in the pursuit of treatment options for cancer.

But the most revolutionary process in medicine is the equalization of power between the patient and his physician. Patients want options. Has your physician offered you choices and guided you toward the best one? Patients want to be well read about their diseases. Has your physician given you resource materials, both written and video? Patients want to keep abreast of new developments. Has your physician told you what's new in the field and what research may benefit you in a few years? Patients want to be part of the medical decision-making process.

Does your physician talk to you and involve you in your own care? Physicians today welcome the chance to step down from their artificial pedestals and become what they once were—trusted friends of a family and servants to the sick. Have you found a physician you respect and call friend?

Perhaps you bought this book hoping it would be an easy-to-follow, all-purpose manual for the prostate. Or perhaps you hope to find that quick, easy, and preferably magical cure for your prostate disorder here in these pages. My friend, I am sorry to disillusion you—there is no such beast.

However, if you seek guidance and information concerning the problems that face the prostate sufferer, then you have indeed found a marvelous sourcebook. For most men, information about the prostate is scarce; men themselves don't like to talk about it openly. The United States government spends $90 million each year educating women about breast cancer, but only $7 million is spent annually educating men about prostate cancer.

Chet Cunningham has written this carefully researched book about the prostate in a friendly and easy-to-understand style. This book brings knowledge from the medical literature to every man who wants to understand the functions and malfunctions of his prostate.

Prostate problems affect men both young and old. We all remember our fathers and grandfathers and the illnesses they suffered. We all have some fear about facing prostate problems because it brings us to the realization that perhaps we, too, are getting older. Or perhaps we don't want to talk about our prostate problems because they may reflect on our sexuality, and we are afraid to admit that anything might be wrong.

What do I hope this book will accomplish? I want every man who reads this book to make it a point of honor to know his own PSA.

I want every man who reads this book to make it a point of honor to persuade one friend or relative to get a yearly digital rectal examination. I want every man who reads this book not to be afraid, but to go out and find a physician who will help him.

I recommend this book highly, not as a substitute for good medical advice, but as a tool for making better, more informed medical choices. This book will be a valuable resource as you become a better partner with your urologist on the patient physician team.

ISRAEL BARKEN, MD, FACS
Board Certified Urologist, San Diego
Assistant Clinical Professor, University of California, San Diego

Fellow, American College of Surgeons
Fellow, American Society for Laser Medicine and Surgery

Introduction

Let's face it, men, the years sneak up on us quickly, far too fast for most of us. It's like the hero in *ON GOLDEN POND* said to his family: "I'm not surprised that I'm eighty years old. But I am surprised that I got here so fast!"

If you're a man over forty years of age, you can't afford to miss reading this book about your prostate. Prostate problems are one of the leading, and often hushed up, ailments in men over forty. The prostate is often where cancer strikes men in their later years.

This book tells you in simple, layman's terms, what your prostate is, where it is positioned, what it does, how it functions and a large variety of ways it can cause problems. We show you what symptoms and behavior patterns to watch for. Remember, these are going to come on slowly and it's always hard to realize there is a change taking place. This book suggests, almost orders you to go see your doctor if you have any of the symptoms of prostate trouble.

This book shows why the problem is occurring,

and when something needs to be done about it. We also include a lot of practical man-to-man suggestions that may be of help to you so you can live with the first and intermediate stages of BPH, Benign Prostatic Hyperplasia, one of the most common prostate problems.

This is not a medical book in any sense of the word. While we have made every effort to be medically exacting and accurate, and have had the manuscript reviewed by a top urologist, the tone and slant of this volume is from one layman to another. No medical term is used without it being explained. You won't need a medical dictionary to understand this book.

It's written to show you some of the problems you may have when you're 40, 50, 60, 70 and 80. Yes, prostate problems can happen to anyone. Remember former President Ronald Reagan had had two prostatic surgeries.

We will be pushing the scientific development "envelope" in the prostate treatment field. We will touch upon all of the latest techniques and surgeries and treatments for the several kinds of prostate troubles including cancer.

We want you to know what's happening to your body, we want to get you to your family doctor or a urologist, and we want you to be aware of the various types of tests and treatments for prostate problems. (*Urologist,* a physician who specializes in the diagnosis and treatment of problems of men and women's urinary tract and the male reproductive system.)

Every man over fifty years of age should have a

PSA blood test once a year to check for any development of cancer of the prostate. This simple blood test shows the amount of prostatic antigen in the bloodstream. This prostatic antigen is a protein antigen produced only by the prostate.

There is a normal amount of PSA in every prostate. As a man's prostate grows, this level will gradually rise. If you have cancer in your prostate, that PSA number increases dramatically and is a signal for your doctor to do further testing to see if you do have cancer of the prostate.

When prostatic cancer is found early, it can usually be caught before it spreads from the prostate to other parts of the body, and the disease can be stopped. Early detection is the key.

How can you get a PSA? Once a year, tell your GP or urologist, or your HMO or other health provider, that you want a PSA test made on your blood. A sample will be drawn and tested, and your doctor will get the results. The PSA level will show your doctor whether or not more tests are needed. Remember your PSA level, and write it down in your permanent records for later comparison.

The PSA test is not infallible, and it sometimes reads positive when it shouldn't. But this is erring on the side of safety. The PSA test is the simplest, least invasive, and best way right now to test your body for the early stages of prostate cancer.

The PSA test will be talked about in more detail later. If you read this book no farther, be sure to have a PSA test. You owe it to yourself and to your wife and your children. Make an appointment with your health provider, your health insurance company, your HMO, or your doctor to have the PSA blood test done.

It doesn't hurt, is noninvasive, and could very well save your life.

Make that doctor's appointment right now!

Notice

This book is not intended to be a substitute for medical advice or treatment of prostate problems. It is an educational and informational book designed to acquaint the average layman with his prostate, its position in the body, its functions, its diseases, conditions and treatments for them. Self diagnosis can be dangerous. If you have a problem with urinating, or think you might have, make an appointment with your family physician, or a urologist, a specialist in this field.

1

What Is My Prostate?

In the male of the species, the prostate is situated directly below the bladder and in front of the inner wall of the rectum. The bladder stores urine produced in the kidneys. A tube going from the bladder to the penis is called the urethra. The urethra passes through the middle of the prostate something like an apple core is in the center of an apple.

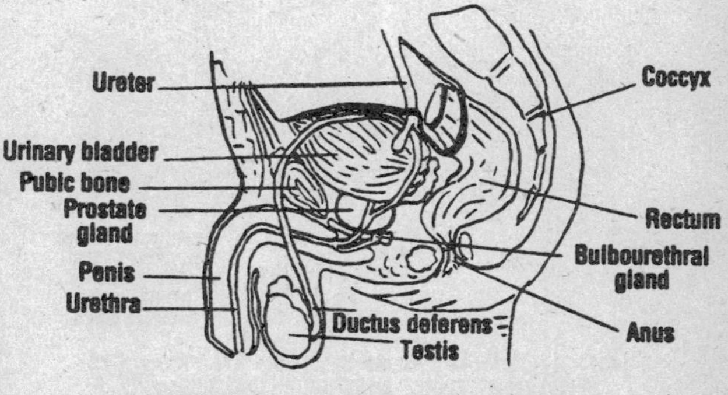

THE GENITOURINARY SYSTEM

The prostate is both muscle and gland, so it's called musculoglandular. It is made up of true prostate tissue and of a harder, fibrous material on the outside called the prostate capsule.

This roughly triangular shaped gland is one to one and a half inches in width, and can weigh between fifteen and twenty grams, depending on the size of the man. That means the prostate gland in most men normally weighs less than an ounce.

When you were born, your prostate was about the size of a medium garden pea and grew gradually. At puberty, the prostate takes a spurt of quick growth. This growth continues at a slower pace until a man is about thirty. At this point the prostate reaches its full adult size.

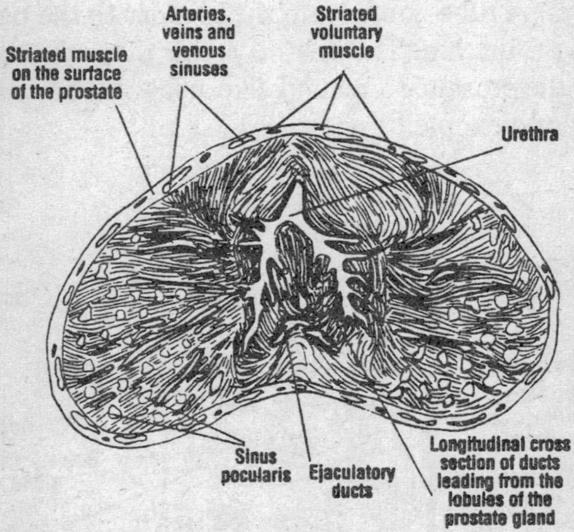

LONGITUDINAL CROSS SECTION OF PROSTATE SHOWING THREE DISTINCT LOBULES AND CENTRAL URETHRAL AREA

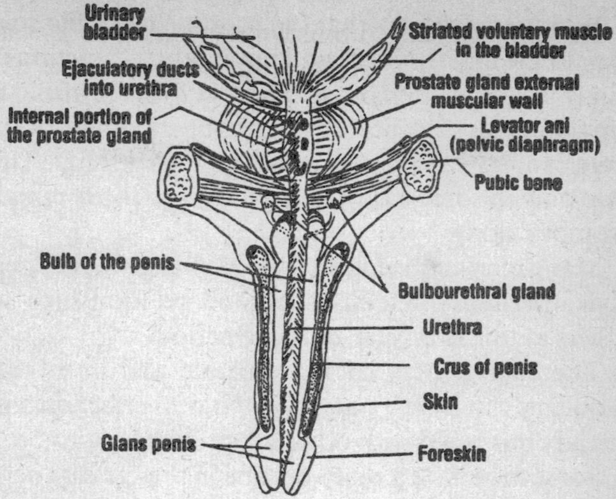

From thirty to fifty years of age, most men's prostates remain about the same size, but after fifty, for some unknown reason, the prostate in most men begins to enlarge. Medical experts say this growth may be the result of a change in the male hormone balance in the system, or it could be some other result of age sneaking up on us that we don't know about yet.

The prostate gland itself is a complex one. It is made up of muscles, glands and fibrous tissues. The many small glands in the prostate are where the fluid is produced that is emptied into the prostatic urethra.

This fluid is injected into the urethra. At the same time the tube that brings the spermatozoa from the testes also emits its product into the urethra. These two fluids, plus one from the seminal vesicles all are combined in the urethra and then ejaculated by the spasmodic contractions of muscles surrounding the urethra.

Which is all to say that the prostate has a big role to play in the male animal, and his ability to function normally in sexual intercourse. So most men are afraid that anything that disrupts the normal operation of the postrate can have an adverse affect on their sex life. This is true only in some cases, and we'll get to those points as we move along.

Many men go through a serious change in life, in lifestyle, perhaps in their work and relationships with others at this fifty-year-old time period.

The enlargement of the prostate and its resulting problems can have a bad psychological effect on a man already burdened with other life problems.

Some men have a sharp decline in their sexual performance about this time. Others might be having work or career problems. A man's wife might be having her own change-of-life difficulties and the children often are drifting away from a close family unit about this time.

When things start to happen to his "water works," and he isn't sure how this will affect his performance in bed, many men become over sensitive about prostate and prostatic problems.

The extent of this enlargement during the fifties and later often is accompanied by three gradually developing habit patterns: there is a decrease in the force and stream of urine. This sometimes is accompanied by a hesitancy to begin urination. Another early symptom that something is wrong is what doctors call nocturia, or simply the need to get up once, twice, or three times a night to urinate.

These minor difficulties are not horrendous, and you can learn to live with them with little disruption of your normal daily activity. Many men live through their fifties and sixties with few of the symptoms of BPH. These letters will be used a lot in this book. They stand for Benign Prostatic Hyperplasia. That simply means a non-cancerous enlargement of the prostate gland.

In the seventies and eighties in most men, more problems can occur and other prostate ailments and dysfunctions can arise. We'll be dealing with them in detail later on.

One expert said that sixty percent of all men over sixty years of age have some BPH, and more than ninety-five percent of men in their eighties have some BPH problems.

What we're saying here is that BPH is simply a factor of older age, like balding heads and weakening muscles. BPH is a fact of life that almost all of us are going to have to learn to live with. The more we can know about it, and the other prostatic problems now, the better we'll be able to cope with it when it becomes serious about hitting us where it hurts.

Other Prostate Disorders

Besides BPH there are several other problems that the prostate can develop which we'll investigate in this book.

One is infectious prostatitis, both acute and chronic. This is an inflammation of the prostate that is common. It can occur at any time from teenage to octagenarian. It is painful and can bring about severe psychological based fears.

Often it seems more serious than it really is and it usually responds well to treatment.

Noninfectious prostatitis includes conditions brought about by sexual activity. Curiously enough this can result from too much sex, or too little, from extreme sexual excitement where there is no ejaculation, as well as prolonged abstinence from intercourse. We'll go into these problems in detail later.

The last disease of the prostate is the most serious and the most frightening to men—prostatic cancer.

Cancer is simply the uncontrolled growth of abnormal cells. In the prostate it is often painless and not quickly detected. Once a problem is suspected, diagnosis is relatively quick and simple. Cancer of the prostate is the second most common cancer in men behind lung cancer. However it's easier to defeat today than it ever has been before.

One out of every eleven men in this country will develop prostate cancer at some time during his life. This is the educated estimation by the American Cancer Society. They say 28,000 men die of prostate cancer each year, but the number would be much lower with a vigorous campaign for early detection.

We'll look into each aspect of prostatic cancer in later chapters.

So, there you have the first look at your prostate. Nothing to go into a panic about, only a small gland with external secretion, that everyone of us should know more about and learn how to live with it and sometimes in spite of it.

Remember that anytime a physician or urologist can catch a problem early, the better he can treat it, and often cure it. Here is a list of prostate trouble symptoms for you to ponder. The symptoms are the same for several different types of prostate troubles. If you have any of these problems, make sure that you see a doctor or urologist quickly. Such a trip just might save your life.

Prostate problem symptoms:

- A slowing of urine stream or force.
- A frequent urge to urinate, most noticed by needing to get up two or three times a night.
- Slowness in starting to urinate. Hesitancy, stopping and starting. A spasm that stops urination.
- Discomfort or pain during urination.
- A sharp pain in pelvic or rectal area.
- Incomplete emptying of the bladder.
- Inability to stop urinating, a continuing dribble.
- Trace or stains of blood in urine.
- Nausea, dizziness or unusual sleepiness.

How can something so small cause so much trouble?

Doctors wish that they knew. The biggest problem is getting men to realize there might be a problem and going to a doctor to find out what it is. Most prostate troubles are not cancerous. One doctor said no more than 30% of all prostatic troubles were the result of cancer.

If it is cancer, your very life could depend on an early diagnosis and treatment.

Most prostate problems and their treatments will not sterilize you or cause impotency or any other sexual performance changes in your current lifestyle. Even the BPH surgery that may result in sterilization is usually not an important factor to a man in his late sixties or seventies. But the chance of finding an early cancer could be lifesaving.

No. We're not trying to scare you. One urologist has

said that men over fifty years of age should get a prostate examination for cancer every time his wife gets a mammogram.

Debunking Some Lies, Myths And Old Wives Tales

This is a good time to start debunking some of the wild stories and myths and gossip that usually makes the rounds about the lowly prostate. Here are a list of the top ten. You may have heard of some more:

1. Prostate surgery always causes a man to become impotent.

This is simply not true. In the past it was more true than it is today, but now there are newer techniques used in surgery that do not disturb the nerve bundles that run on either side of the prostate. These nerves control a man's ability to have an erection and intercourse. In cancer surgery, doctors have learned to remove the prostate usually without damaging these nerve bundles. However, some patients still suffer impotency. In the BPH surgery, only five percent of patients suffer any impotency.

2. An enlarged prostate, BPH, is a leading cause of prostate cancer.

Absolutely not. The enlargement of the prostate is in no way connected to the development of prostatic cancer. The cause of the enlargement is not known, but the cause of cancer is and the two are not linked. This myth may have come about because during some surgeries for the relief of BPH, the prostate is found to be cancerous when it had not been so diagnosed before. This actually can be one of the hidden benefits of such surgery.

3. Prostate surgery automatically sterilizes you.

In one half to two-thirds of the patients who have prostatic surgery where some or all of the prostate is removed, the normal course of the semen and other fluids usually ejaculated is disrupted. The fluid takes the course of least resistance and flows upward into the bladder instead of down the urethra and out the penis. To a man 60 or 65 this is usually not so important. However if children are wanted, the semen can be captured from urination soon after the orgasm and used for artificial insemination.

4. Prostate problems turn a man into a wimp.

If this happens it isn't the result of the prostate problems. There is no loss of manhood, physical or psychological from any of the prostatic problems. There may be psychological side effects by various individuals, but these are mental in nature and could be casued by any number of reasons.

5. Prostate disorders are embarrassing to talk about because they mean a man is oversexed and having sex far too often.

A pure fantasy. Prostate problems and their treatments should not be embarrassing to talk about. Indeed a woman should realize an intelligent and understanding attitude toward prostate testing and evaluation, could save her husband's life.

6. Orgasm for the man after prostate surgery isn't the same, isn't satisfying.

Simply not true. In case after case, the men report that the feeling at the time of orgasm and ejaculation is unchanged from what it was before surgery. Whether the ejaculation fluids go back into the bladder or out the penis, the feeling is exactly the same for the man. If there is a change, it is psychological and unfounded.

7. "Damn, man. Your sex life is over after BPH surgery."

Again, not factual. Any man's sex life changes as he gets older. In his sixties and seventies a man has sex less frequently than when he was twenty. For at least ninety-five percent, a man's sex life will be the same after BPH surgery as it was before. For the other five percent, there will be some problems with impotency—but that can be dealt with.

8. Incontinence is an automatic result of BPH surgery.

Researchers show us that only four percent of all BPH surgeries will result in the patients having trouble retaining their urine. That's twenty-five to one odds, not bad.

9. There are lots of over the counter remedies that will cure my prostate without surgery.

By the end of 1990, the FDA took all such advertised remedies off the market. Previously the Postal Inspectors had closed down dozens of mail order houses who sold them. We will talk about the compounds in these products. Many people believe they are effective in reducing symptoms of BPH. Most do not say they can cure prostatic problems.

10. Prostate is a dirty word and a gentleman never mentions it in mixed company.

Ridiculous. In this more enlightened age, when women are encourged to examine their breasts for lumps, men must be encouraged and badgered into having at least yearly prostate examinations. The best way to do this is through education, and talking about the problem. Talking to the wives of the target men is often the most effective method.

Now, let's move on to an in-depth look at the ailment that affects nearly all older men, BPH.

2

Benign Prostatic Hyperplasia . . . BPH

What Is BPH

Benign Prostatic Hyperplasia, sometimes called Hypertrophy, is the medical way of saying that the prostate gland has enlarged. In early stages this enlargement may not cause any problems. As it enlarges more and more with a man's increasing age, it may squeeze the urethra smaller and smaller.

This reduces the force and size of your urine stream, and if left untreated, BPH could lead to the closure of the urethra resulting in severe sickness and even death.

Doctors say that in BPH the glandular tissue within the prostate capsule enlarges, grows, and no one seems to know why it happens or how to prevent or stop this growth.

This is a benign growth. That means it is not cancerous, it does not spread to other parts of the body or attack other tissues or cells. If it were malignant, as in cancer of the prostate, it would destroy and attack other tissue or cells and spread.

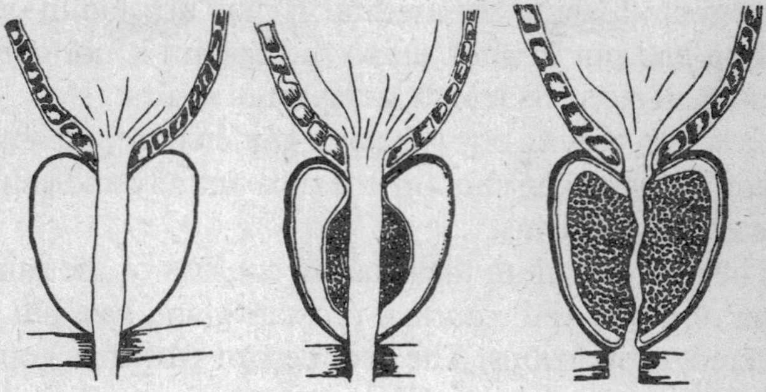

In the drawings here, notice how the urethra is fully open in the first one. It passes through the prostate allowing normal flow of urine from the bladder through the urethra and out the penis.

In the second drawing, the darker growth of benign tissue has begun and already has taken the bulge out of the urethra. In the third drawing, the BPH tissue has almost closed the tube the urine must pass through, making urination extremely difficult and bringing on all sorts of BPH symptoms and problems.

We come back to the apple example. Your prostate is like an apple with the core taken out. Through the core goes the urethra. The size of the urethra may begin to shrink when the prostate starts to enlarge when most men are about forty to forty-five. Often by the time a man is in his fifties he's noticing some changes in his urination pattern.

It is just outside the urethra where the benign growth of the prostatic tissue begins, and it usually grows in both directions, which at once impacts the size of the urethra.

The growth of the tissue usually is not uniform or consistent all along the urethra. It may develop in one section and not in another, so the urethra is not compressed all along its length, at least not at first.

However, as with any tube or a garden hose, pressure at any one spot can shut off the tube entirely and cause all sorts of problems.

The new growth in the prostate consists of the same types of tissue as the normal prostate gland has, but in different proportions. The new, benign growth is going to have more of the glandular type of tissue.

The new growth in the prostate usually develops in both an inward and outward direction, toward the urethra and toward the exterior of the gland. When it grows outward it compresses the normal prostatic tissue against the sturdy outer capsule of the prostate.

When this outer growth takes place in the two lobes of the prostate nearest the rectum, a specialist can feel this with a digital examination. The outward growth does not narrow the urethra so there would be none of the usual BPH symptoms.

In most cases, however, when there is an outward growth of the tissue, it also grows toward the inside as well. Now we get the narrowing of the urethra over the years, and the normal symptoms of BPH.

The prostate has several sections, and digital examination can touch only the back part of the prostate. The sections that can't be felt can harbor benign or malignant growth. This is one of the reasons for other tests for prostatic cancer that we'll explain in detail later.

Symptoms of an Enlarged Prostate

Do you have any of the symptoms of an enlarged prostate? Here is a list of those problems that relate directly to BPH. Study the list critically. Have you experienced any of them?

- A slowing of your urinary stream and its force.
- A slowness to begin urination. You say "start now," but it may be a few seconds before your stream begins.
- A problem with stopping urination. You tighten the muscles to stop the flow or to prevent any more, but you get a series of continuing dribbles.
- A sensation that your bladder is not completely empty when it should be.
- Frequent urination. You may not notice this during the day, especially if you're near a bathroom. But at night this is much more evident. Doctors call this nocturia, and it may get you up two, three, four times a night.
- In extreme cases, urinary retention—when you simply can't urinate. The discomfort and pain can be tremendous.
- Nausea, dizziness, unusual sleepiness brought on if retention has caused kidney damage.

A Simple Test You Can Give Yourself

Below is a chart with the symptoms listed above. Some of them are worded differently. At the top are the points to be given for each symptom and its severity. Along the left side are the symptoms.

POINTS	0	1	2	3	4
STREAM	Normal	Variable		Weak	Dribbling
VOIDING	No Strain		Abdominal strain or Credé		
HESITANCY	None			Yes	
INTERMITTENCY	None			Yes	
BLADDER EMPTYING	Don't know or Complete	Variable	Incomplete	Single retention	Repeated retention
INCONTINENCE			Yes (Including Terminal Dribbling)		
URGE	None	Mild	Moderate	Severe (Incontinence)	
NOCTURIA	0 - 1	2	3 - 4	>4	
DIURIA	q > 3h	q2 - 3h	q1 - 2h	q < 1h	

TOTAL SCORE

Intermittency means that your stream starts, stops and starts again once or more before you feel empty. Incontinence means that you can't stop urinating when you want to, or you dribble, or pass some water when you don't want to.

Diuria, means how often your need to urinate during the day. Zero points for three hours or more and 3 points for the need to void each hour during the day.

Mark down what you think your symptoms are. If your score reaches 10 or more, you should probably see your doctor soon about the chances you have BPH.

What Causes BPH?

No one knows what causes BPH. Just why the prostate starts to enlarge itself in the forty to fifty male years is not understood.

There are two significant factors in this mystery that have been tied down by medical research over the years.

One is that a man who has been surgically or hormonally castrated, eliminating the male hormone from his body, never develops an enlarged prostate.

The other uncontested fact is that the onset of BPH is started only with the passage of time.

Castration at an early age to eliminate BPH is a totally unthinkable idea. The other alternative, death at an early age is equally ridiculous as a prevention of BPH.

Which leaves medical science still in kindergarten when it comes to determining the cause of BPH and the chances of scientifically developing a preventive drug or routine and this stops any work on a cure.

Many medical studies have been made in an effort to isolate some other common factor in BPH patients. So far all of these human factors have been ruled out: specific blood types, coronary heart disease, celibacy, hypertension, use of alcohol or tobacco, industrial and environmental conditions.

One constant has been determined: By the age of sixty years, fifty percent of all men will have, to some degree, an enlarged prostate whether or not it is bothering them. By the time American men reach their eightieth birthday, only five out of one hundred will not have BPH.

After broad studies involving Asian men, it was determined that as a group they had fewer cases of BPH and prostatic cancer. However Asian men who moved to the US for a period of time had a significantly increased rate of both BPH and prostatic cancer.

Since Asians typically have had a low cholesterol and low red meat diet, it is speculated that diet may have a larger impact on BPH and prostatic cancer than had been previously thought. With the current wave of anti-cholesterol and anti-fat foods including the campaign against red meat, American men could be experiencing a lower rate of BPH and prostatic cancer in the future.

Is a man's sex life in any way connected with the cause of BPH or prostatic cancer? A man's sexual life appears to have no bearing whatsoever on the development of BPH or cancer of the prostate. However, sudden surges in sexual activity, or sudden celibacy often does affect the prostate. These situations will be discussed in a later section.

So What Happens to Me Next?

Let's say that you're reading this book in the first place because you had some questions about your general health, or your urination, or your prostate, and after reading the list of symptoms, bingo! you have three of the symptoms.

Let's say that you have a hesitancy to start to urinate, you have a noticeably reduced stream, and you've been getting up about three A.M. every night to urinate.

What should you do next?

Pick up the phone and get an appointment with your family doctor or call a urologist. It's time you found out just what's going on and how serious your BPH really is.

Your next move is to have an examination by a medical professional or a specialist. Just how does a doctor examine you for possible BPH or other prostatic troubles?

The first exam will be the digital one. Since the prostate is right next to the rectum, it can be palpitated. In this slightly uncomfortable digital exam, the doctor is checking to see if your prostate feels enlarged. He is also finding out if there are any hard spots or lumps or nodes on the two lobes he can touch.

The healthy prostate is smooth, elastic and about the size of a walnut. If there is BPH, the prostate will still feel about the same way but it will be obviously enlarged.

Most urologists say that a digital examination can't confirm 100 percent the presence of BPH. They point out, however that with such an exam showing the prostate is soft and rubbery, that there is an enlargement outward of two of the prostate lobes, and that the patient reports three symptoms of BPH, there is sufficient evidence to diagnose BPH.

In the fast paced routines in many HMO's these days, a patient with these workups may very well be told he has BPH, be shown a video tape concerning the problem, and be told what to do to make living with the condition easier.

He'll be told that in the early stages of BPH, a patient is not a good candidate for surgery or other regular treatment. Rather he will be put on a "maintenance" program where he is checked by a urologist yearly for any progress of the condition.

Many doctors and urologists say this is the proper course of care. They show histories of men in their fifties who have been on maintenance care for ten, even fifteen years before the prostate enlarged to such a point that surgery or one of the new treatments was necessary.

Another test your urolgist may make is a peak flow test. This can be done with an instrument that will record the flow much as the charts below show.

The first chart shows a more or less normal rate of flow with a peak about half way through and stopping quickly. The lower chart shows a much weaker flow and over twice to three times the length of time. This usually means some serious blockage in the urethra and the urologist will want to follow up with other tests.

Some urologists use a stop watch and a timed urination into a glass to approximate the same results.

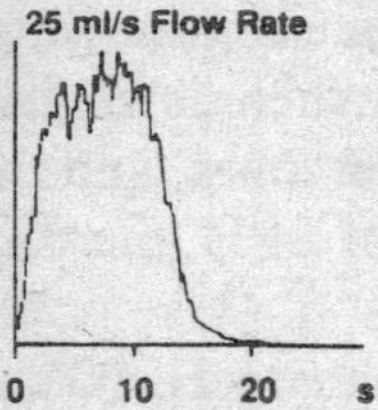

Results of UROFLOWMETRY

T100	17	s
TQ	17	s
TQmax	7	s
Qmax	24.0	ml/s
Qave	14.1	ml/s
Vcomp	247	ml

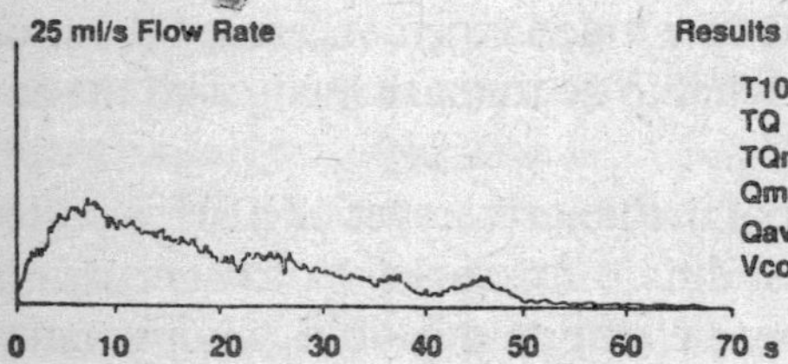

Results of UROFLOWMETRY

T100	60	s
TQ	51	s
TQmax	8	s
Qmax	10.2	ml/s
Qave	4.1	ml/s
Vcomp	211	ml

Are Any Other Tests Available?

Yes, there are several other tests that urologists can use with the prostate. Some of these are used when prostatic cancer is suspected.

However, since some ten percent of all surgery done to relieve BPH results in finding early stages of prostatic cancer development, some men ask for additional tests. They want to make sure that their prostate is not cancerous as well as having BPH.

These tests in effect become Negative Testing, to assure the patient that there is no cancer in the prostate lobes that can't be felt by the digital exam.

The PSA Prostate Cancer Test

Another test to determine if the patient may have cancer of the prostate is the Prostate Specific Antigen or PSA test. It has been developed in the past three or four years and many men don't know about it yet.

It is the best nonintrusive system yet that may show the presence of prostate cancer in even the smallest amount.

The PSA is a simple blood evaluation. The test should be drawn before any manipulation or touching of the prostate is done by a surgeon's gloved finger that is part of most thorough adult male physical exams. Such probing upsets the normal antigen level in the prostate and results in a false reading.

If cancer strikes the prostate, it manufactures increased amounts of antigen in a reaction to the cancer. These antigens are thought to react to a number of different prostate cancers. Every prostate has a normal antigen level. However, studies have shown a definite correlation between the PSA and the volume of cancer in the prostate. If only a very few cancer cells are present in the prostate, the antigen level will be raised only a little.

If the prostate is heavily infected with cancer, the antigen level may go from a norm of either 2 or 4 (depending on the type test) up into the 200s.

The PSA test is calibrated two different ways. One system uses a 2 level as normal. The other uses a 4 level as normal. As the prostate grows in size, the normal amount of antigen level may increase. A reading on the 4 point scale of a 4.8 antigen level, for example, would reflect that growth, and not indicate any cancer, especially if the patient has an enlarged prostate and BPH.

Some doctors say the PSA test can give false indications about cancer in the prostate. The fact is, such a blood test should be only *one* of the elements in a complete examination if a patient is thought to have prostate cancer. Not every elevated PSA means cancer is present.

The antigen level indication of some cancer can be confirmed or disproved with an ultrasound rectal probe to present a complete picture of the prostate on a screen.

Why is the PSA test so important?

It is nonintrusive. Many men simply will not allow a doctor to do a rectal digital exam of the prostate. They refuse, and no argument will convince them that their life could be at stake.

The simple blood test gives the doctor and the patient's wife and family some leverage to use if the PSA shows a serious elevation. The results of a PSA test can convince the patient that more tests are needed, including the ultrasound imaging.

The PSA test can detect minute quantities of cancer cells in the prostate and do it long before a regular digital examination could pick up any hard, cancerous lumps. This means the PSA test is ideal for catching the cancer early. As with any cancer, the earlier it is diagnosed, the better the chances of its successful treatment.

Early detection means the cancer has not had a chance to metastasize or spread into the lymph glands, or into other body parts such as hip or knee joints, the spine, or the brain. When the cancer spreads this way before it is detected, it is usually not possible to cure it.

The PSA test should also be used as a method of follow-up after prostate cancer surgery to be sure all cancer cells were removed. It can then be used at six-month intervals with the surgery patient to see if there is any recurrence of the cancer.

Early detection is the key. Early prostate cancer detection by the PSA test or any other means is the best way to stop prostate cancer from ending your life.

Ultrasound Testing

One of the newer tools of the urologist is the use of ultrasound. This is sometimes called sonography. It simply uses high-frequency sound waves to examine a specific part of the body and make a record of it.

The record can be a sonogram on special film or on paper, or the whole process can be recorded on video tape for critical examination later, and as a record for comparison later of any growth or changes or condition of the examined areas.

The test is quick, simple and painless. A wand instrument called a transducer is passed back and forth over the area being examined. The wand transmits sound waves that are echoed back to it much like a radar does.

The echoes are electronically transmitted to the recording or viewing device.

When examining the bladder and prostate with ultrasound, the bladder needs to be full of urine. Then the test is repeated after the man has urinated to see what urine remains in the bladder.

Ultrasound is becoming more and more popular with urologists and most hospitals have it available. Many urologists now have ultrasound capability as a part of their office equipment for use when needed.

Another use of the ultrasound system is called a transrectal probe. It can be used in conjunction with a surface sonogram.

Many urologists recommend the transrectal. In this test a probe, covered with a rubber balloon which is then filled with water, is inserted into the rectum. This creates an ultrasonic image of the prostate and bladder area that can be recorded and at the same time viewed on a screen.

Some urologists say the transrectal sonogram will show many false leads that are not really cancer. Others say it is a fine method to determine if there is an area that seems to be a cancer and calls for more investigation.

Magnetic Resonance Imaging

MRI is an expensive testing method that is painless and quick and can produce a three-dimensional cross section of any part of the body. Users say it is even more detailed than the images produced by a CAT scan.

This test is non-invasive and has no radiation. It uses

radio waves in a magnetic field to produce the picture. This test is almost always done in a large hospital.

These days, all testing is expensive. If you have the three-symptom case of BPH, and the digital examination has led to a diagnosis by the physician that as far as he can feel there is no sign of cancer, then it is up to you to decide if you wish to have any more tests to prove to yourself that you are cancer free. Some of these tests, such as ultrasound, are not covered by some of the insurance companies.

One patient was adamant about receiving more tests. He had the three symptom BPH, felt fine, but had a friend who was dying of prostatic cancer. It was well worth it to him to have a $200 sonogram taken that showed no noticeable sign of cancer in his prostate. He was still concerned about the 10 percent of BPH surgery that reveals prostatic cancer. His doctor pointed out to him that such surgeries were performed at a much later point in life than he was. The doctor also said that such BPH problems were much farther developed and had been growing for a greater length of time than his had.

He understood the logic of the urologist. He had been living with his BPH for only about five years. He left the office but a week later called for another appointment. When he came in he said he wanted to take the two blood tests that could reveal the presence of cancer in the prostate, the PAP and PSA tests. Both were made and both showed up negative. Another sign that he did not have prostatic cancer.

The patient was now convinced. He told the urologist that he was not showing disrespect for his qualifications or his skills, but he wanted a little more assurance that he didn't have cancer than the simple digital examination by the doctor.

What Problems Can Extreme Prostate Enlargement Cause?

Silent Prostatism. Sometimes the prostate will enlarge and there are none of the usual symptoms. The urethra continues to close but somehow the man simply doesn't realize the problem or decides that he's just getting old and the "water works" sometimes doesn't work right for him.

If this condition builds and builds, more and more urine can be left in the bladder that can't be expelled in urination. This can result in a serious problem. The patient will become excessively tired and feel weak, he will be irritable and could suddenly collapse or even lapse into a coma.

When large amounts of urine are left in the bladder and it isn't strong enough to expel the liquid through a narrowing urethra, serious damage can occur. This can lead to a serious backflow pressure of the urine on the kidneys. At the most serious, such a problem can cause kidney failure and a quick death.

In cases like this the patient needs to get to a hospital quickly so a catheter can be used to drain the bladder. With the emptying of the bladder, the patient will feel much better almost at once. Then the doctors will watch to see if any permanent damage was done to the kidneys and if so what additional treatment might be needed.

Depending on the seriousness of the situation, the

patient's normal kidney function should come back after a week to three months. At that time the prostate should be checked for size to see if prostate surgery or some other treatment is required.

Congestion Of The Prostate

Sometimes after normal BPH symptoms in a patient, an urologist will find only a moderately enlarged prostate but one that is mildly congested. There often is no sign of infection. Typically there might be a minor amount of urine that can't be drained from the bladder during urination.

Often there will be some form of obstruction at the bladder outlet which also restricts bladder emptying.

At this point there is no major problem for the patient and he would be put on a maintenance program to have his prostate checked regularly.

As the prostate grows and the bladder muscles are forced to work harder and harder to push the urine through the narrowing urethra, the bladder can become fatigued. In some cases the bladder will simply quit functioning and urine buildup occurs in the bladder.

This can form a place where bacteria can grow and multiply rapidly. When this happens the patient feels a burning pain when he urinates. Sometimes the urine will have a bad odor and traces of blood can show in the urine.

A danger here is urinary infection, which is usually signalled in the patient by a burning sensation when urinating, chills or fever and the intensification of his regular BPH symptoms.

Here, as in other early symptoms of BPH, the patient may go for several years without any more serious problems than his minor BPH problems.

On the other hand the congestion may increase, and if this happens the patient's urologist may suggest a prostate massage. Here the prostate is massaged digitally through the rectum and the congested fluid is expelled. This makes the heaviness vanish and a more normal life returns.

The urologist may suggest that a patient have regular prostate massages to relieve the congestion. Or it may be relieved by regular ejaculations through intercourse or masturbation.

Some urologists never recommend repeated prostatic massages. But all suggest in situations like this that the patient should avoid long periods of exposure to intense cold weather, should avoid most spicy foods, should sharply reduce the use of alcoholic beverages, should avoid antihistamines, and they recommend the patient to take warm baths often.

Any shift or intensifying or change in symptoms of the BPH should be reported to the patient's physician or urologist at once.

Acute Urine Retention

In this busy, busy world of ours, many men are working so hard and going so fast that they don't take time for regular physical checkups. Some never think about prostate problems until it's almost too late.

Again the symptoms of BPH can slip up on a busy man. He simply figures that by sixty-three he should be urinating more often and he's heard other men talk about needing to get up at night once or twice. He thinks nothing of it.

Then one day he needs to urinate but can't. He stands there waiting and then straining but he can't pass even a few drops and he's hurting like crazy. Soon the pain is so agonizing that he calls his doctor or rushes down to a hospital emergency room to find out what's the matter.

A catheter drains the urine from the distended bladder and relieves the problem. Some patients with acute urine retention might be holding as much as a quart of urine. Most patients will look much better within minutes and feel fine in an hour or so.

A sudden attack of acute urine retention can happen to almost any man who has some obstruction already in his urethra. There are also conditions that can bring on such attacks.

Prolonged exposure to the cold, especially if you are not used to it can sometimes bring on such an attack. Drinking alcohol by someone not used to it. The sudden use of antihistamines is also a culprit in this case.

Such an attack is usually enough for the patient to have his prostate checked critically by an urologist who will advise him if any treatment or surgery is needed— as well as suggestions about how to prevent such an attack in the future.

So, there is your primer on BPH, its symptoms and some details about the problems it brings up. Now, there is a way to live with these problems during that time when the doctor recommends no major treatment is needed. We'll look at that in the next chapter.

3

How To Cope With Early BPH

Living with the early stages of an enlarged prostate isn't all that hard:

This is true. Remember, you had BPH for eight to ten years before it caused you any problems at all. You might have had some mild symptoms for another two or three years before you realized it and found out what was causing them. Now you know.

Now is no time to panic. So these problems caused by BPH are a small inconvenience, they are something you can learn to live with. The alternative is not a happy thought.

Let's go back to our typical case history. This gentleman is the one who is sixty years old and has the three most minor of BPH symptoms: a brief hesitancy when urinating, a slower, less forceful stream, and he usually gets up once a night to urinate.

The secret here is that you *know* what the cause is of these minor problems, which means you can learn to manage them. You have managed a lot of things in your life, right? First the other kids in your family, then a wife, then your own kids, then that business and all the people you had under you. Compared to that, managing early BPH is a breeze.

First the worry. The experts say again and again that BPH is not cancer, has no connection with prostate cancer, does not lead to cancer and is an entirely separate ailment. So get that out of your mind.

You don't have prostate cancer, it's only BPH.

Urologists fight this misconception all the time and gradually they're winning. They point out that cancer of the prostate is almost always on the *outside* of the prostate lobes. The enlarged prostate grows *inward and outward*. There is absolutely no casual relationship between the two.

Now, one more concern with prostate cancer. When surgery is needed for BPH, usually at a much later time than in a man's fifties or early sixties, there is a finding that about ten percent of the BPH prostates will be found to have a cancer.

Remember, cancer can strike any part of the body at any time in life. It has no connection to BPH. When these cancers are found they are not in the usual places where they could be easily diagnosed during your regular BPH exams. So in reality the BPH surgery is a stroke of luck since most of these cancers are just beginning and are caught quickly so they can be eradicated more easily.

So, from here on we don't worry about BPH causing or being tied in with prostate cancer in any way. Clear?

Urologists point out that the minor symptoms of BPH, often the initial ones, may be the only troubles a man suffers with BPH for as much as ten to fifteen years. That means you shouldn't even be thinking about or concerned with any worry about prostate surgery or other treatment now. Dump it right out of your computer memory hard disc. Why worry about something that isn't going to happen for ten to fifteen years? You'll have plenty of time to fret and stew about it and discuss it with your urologist when the time comes. By then some even better treatments undoubtedly will be developed.

Concentrate on today, and how to make your life pleasant and interesting and fulfilling, *right now!* in spite of BPH.

We know that there is no "cure" for BPH. You can't take a pill and like a headache your BPH will just go away. It isn't that kind of a problem. Even with our miracle modern medical cures, there is nothing even on the drawing boards that will magically cure BPH. So we practice positive thinking and forget about that and move on to areas of behavior that we can and should do something about.

Plain old fashioned horse-sense. With the decline of the horse as the basic transportation unit of Americans, not much is heard anymore about horse-sense. Too bad. Horse-sense has shaken down to "common sense," which is almost as good.

For example, it makes no sense to drink two gallons of water a day when you know you're going to have to urinate most of that water the same day. Don't overload your urinary system. The less you drink the less you'll have to urinate.

Don't carry this to extremes. You need water, fluids, to survive. But there is a happy medium. Some doctors say a man should drink eight, eight ounce glasses of water a day. That's half a gallon. Actually what they mean is that the body should intake that much fluid a day: coffee, water, milk, soup, colas, juice, any fluid should count.

Many other doctors say this is much more fluid than the average man needs. Your body will tell you when it wants a drink. As a common sense living-with-BPH, start cutting down on your fluids a little at a time. You'll be urinating less, but still enough. Talk to your urologist or doctor about this and find out what the *minimum* daily need is for intake fluids for a man of your size and activity. It may be much less than you suspect.

If you do manual labor in the hot sun all day, you'll need more water than if you're in an air-conditioned office where you work on a computer. Your doctor will be able to help you here.

Time Your Fluid Intake

If nocturia bothers you, and you're getting up three times a night to urinate, try limiting your fluid intake in the evening. One doctor suggested not to drink any fluids for four hours before retiring. That way your body will have processed your fluids, and passed them well before your sleeping time.

Using a modified system such as this (some men have one small drink at dinner and nothing after that) many

BPH patients can cut to once their nocturnal urination. Now that is a real blessing if you can go from three risings to only one a night. This is a prime example of how you can manage your own life to reduce the interference of BPH with your normal activities.

Alcohol And Beer

You knew this was coming. Alcohol is not good for the human body. Alcohol is especially not good for men with BPH.

"Hell, give up beer and a few shots of bourbon and maybe a highball or two? Damn, I'd rather die!" Such typical comments by moderate and heavy drinkers is often answered with the assurance of: "You will die and probably sooner than you expected to."

For years some urologists have said that alcohol irritates the prostate. It also can cause serious problems with the liver. Some of the flavorings in alcohol can affect the prostate to such a degree that it can cause a kind of chronic prostatitis

For a man with even early BPH, the sudden or overuse of alcohol can bring on a surprise attack of acute retention of urine. This condition results in a desperate need to urinate but it is impossible. A quick trip to a doctor's office or the emergency room of a hospital for catheterization and draining the bladder follows.

Good old common sense dictates that a man with even early BPH should seriously consider his consumption of alcohol and its relation to his prostatic condition. At this point many men simply don't want to take the risk or stand the pain and problems associated with alcohol and BPH and stop drinking.

Beer drinkers will be furious, but the pint-in, pint-out and the much used bathrooms at bars and taverns, indicate that it is well known that beer drinking is immediately followed by voluminous urination.

Here common sense leaps up again. Beer drinking in the afternoon may be easily tolerated by some men, but not by others. Late night beer drinking will almost surely trigger two or three additional night time trips to the bathroom that otherwise could have been avoided.

If you insist on drinking beer, use a little common sense so it doesn't trigger more unpleasant BPH reactions.

Coffee, Colas And Caffeine

Yes, caffeine is the big tiger on your back here. Caffeine is a stimulant to the urinary tract: it makes you urinate more and more frequently. For most well people this is no problem, not even a minor inconvenience. Over the years your body will adapt to the added caffeine.

But when you have BPH, it's different. You don't need any more stimulation in your urinary tract. Neither do you need any more volume.

The BPH coffee drinker who normally goes through twelve, eight ounce cups of coffee a day is going to have a much harder time living with his urinary tract, than the non-coffee drinker, or even the man who drinks twelve, eight ounces of non-caffeine fluids a day.

Ounce for ounce, coffee and tea contain twice the amount of caffeine that regular cola drinks do. Of course now most of the colas come in caffeine free types as well. This is one place where you can have your cola and not your caffeine.

In the same manner, there are many caffeine free coffee brands now on the market.

If you want to manage your body with a little more "smarts" give the caffeine free drinks a test in your own bathroom. You'll probably be pleasantly surprised when you make the test.

Oh, the "Principle of the single differential." When you make any of these intake tests, try to do everything else the same, except for the item you're testing. If you have two differentials (variables) in your life style, you won't be able to tell which one made the difference, if there is a difference. It's an old principle from the physical sciences but it works.

If you drink caffeine fluids, take the test. Try the caffeine free types for a week, doing nothing else different. One BPH patient said it cut his nocturia risings down from two a night to one. After a few weeks you'll even forget what the caffeine laced drink tasted like.

Don't forget that many of the current pain pills for headaches, colds and hay fever also contain caffeine. While these aren't taken often, you might look for some that don't have caffeine in them, such as the ibuprofen medications.

BPH and Over-the-Counter Drugs

One small warning about BPH and over-the-counter or prescription drugs. There are over a hundred medications out there in the pharmacist's shelves that can conflict with and actually make your BPH condition worse.

Whenever you get any medication from a GP or your family doctor or other nonurologist, make sure that he or she understands that you have a continuing BPH problem and that you should be given none of the 100 drugs that should not be used by BPH sufferers.

The drug could be for any condition. Doctors have a computer that will show any drug conflict with other *drugs,* but they don't show a conflict with BPH. Most urologists have a list of the medications that shouldn't be used.

Many pharmacists can tell you if a drug is counterindicated for men with prostate trouble.

One man with BPH was having trouble with his throat. The doctor said he had a postnasal drip and prescribed Enomine, a decongestant.

The man took the two pills a day and soon his urine stream almost vanished and urination became extremely difficult. A call to the druggist revealed that Enomine should not be used by men with prostate trouble. The GP who prescribed it didn't know or didn't check the man's chart to see that he had BPH.

Check with your doctor before using any drug to see that it won't exacerbate prostate problems.

Plan It Out Ahead

There are other ways to live more comfortably with your BPH.

- A long car trip. Plan where you're going to stop. Most car rides tend to stimulate the urinary tract. This may be partly due to nervous tension if you're the driver. Figure out where you can stop at least every two hours.

This will allow you to gas up, have a snack and use the bathroom. Some patients with BPH say sometimes on car trips they have been stuck in big cities where there were no filling stations, and by the time they found one they nearly tore the door off the men's room to get inside.

- Going to a scary or suspenseful movie? Again nervous tension can increase the need to urinate. Performers get this problem before they go on. A really wild movie can do the same thing to most men. Try to use the bathroom before the movie starts. As a precaution, don't buy a large cola drink to go along with your popcorn.

Remember "a pint in, a pint out," and often the "pint out" part won't wait until the movie is over.

- Let's say you waited too long, your whole crotch is burning and throbbing and you have to urinate so bad you're almost upset to your stomach. When you at last get to a bathroom, try for the toilet stall. Simply close the door, drop your pants and sit down.

No one seems to know why, but sitting down to urinate relaxes some muscles or the sphincter muscle, or something, and it makes urination at these difficult times much easier. At stress times like this, many BPH patients say it's taken them five minutes of standing at a urinal or at the bathroom at home before they can get even a drop of urine out.

Spasming of muscles seems to be relaxed, and the whole system simply works easier and much faster in these stress situations, if you can sit down and bend forward toward your knees.

At this point who cares why it works, it does and will

work any time you have trouble getting a urine flow started as well. Don't fight it, just try it!

Coping With Your BPH

You've known that you've been living with your BPH for what—a year, three years? You're a short timer. Most urologists have had literally thousands of years of experience with BPH through their patients. Your doctor may have a dozen little hints and helps like those above that have worked for hundreds of his BPH patients. No, these are not big dramatic findings that can be reported in the New England Journal of Medicine or the Journal of the American Medical Association.

However, your own doctor or urologist may have a small gold mine of tips and hints that he's picked up over the years to make a big difference in how you can live easier and more comfortably with early and more advanced stages of BPH.

The next time you're in his office, ask him if he has any of these little gems of BPH trivia advice that might just fit some problem that you've been having. The best advice is: Always go to the expert: talk to your urologist.

4

Non Major-Surgical BPH Treatments

Remember our typical early BPH patient example? Well your clock has swept around and you're now 63, your minor BPH symptoms are more severe. You can't get through a night without getting up three or four times to urinate. Everytime you wake up you leap out of bed and rush to the bathroom.

During the day you've had to hold up a board meeting while you went to the toilet. You can't take a car drive of more than an hour without stopping. On your business flights you always get an aisle seat so you can hurry to the cramped convenience two or three times during a flight.

Besides that, sometimes it hurts like outrageous sin.

So, you go back to see your urologist. For the past eight years he's been "monitoring" your BPH. At every examination he assures you that there are no hard lumps or irregular growth of the two side prostate lobes. He says that means you probably don't have prostatic cancer.

What happens next? You want some relief, you want to feel better and be able to lead a more normal life. It's a quality of life situation you're talking about and you want some help, now!

Your urologist agrees and the two of you sit down to talk about the possible ways that your situation can be eased. You realize that once the prostate starts to grow, nothing we know of now will stop it, except total sterilization. That's out. What other remedies are there?

The Balloon Method

One of the new treatments now getting wider acceptance is the use of a balloon. Urologists have borrowed this technique from the heart surgeons. The physician inserts a small tube about the size of spaghetti into the urethra. On the far end of the tube is an un-inflated balloon.

When the balloon is in the proper position in the urethra within the enlarged prostate, the physician inflates the balloon. This inflation is held for different lengths of time. Some urologists use a ten minute period of pressure by the balloon within the urethra to force the urethra to expand back to its original position.

This forces the prostate tissues outward. In some cases the outer casing of the prostate is "cracked" or broken to allow the enlarged prostatic tissue to move in that direction and eliminate the pressure on the urethra.

Just who first developed this technique is not

known, but Dr. Flavio Castaneda, a radiologist at St. Francis Medical Center at the University of Illinois in Peoria, is one of the pioneers in the use of this new technique. He says that seventy-five percent of the BPH patients he has used the balloon treatment on have been symptom free for up to three years after the treatment.

In another part of the country, more than 60 patients have been treated with the balloon dilation method at the University of Minnesota.

For eighty percent of these patients the urination problem was eliminated or significantly eased. This was for patients with enlargement of the side lobes of the prostate. When the narrowing of the urethra was because of enlargement of the middle lobe, the success rate dropped to thirty to forty percent.

Dr. Israel Barken, a urologist in San Diego, California, has been using the balloon treatment.

He says for this procedure the patient is tranquilized and the urethra is numbed with a local anesthetic. Then a thin, flexible tube with a balloon on the tip is inserted into the urethra and guided to the narrowed portion. The balloon is then inflated. He says he uses a time of about 20 minutes. This is an outpatient treatment and no hospitalization is needed. If the patient wants the procedure done in the office or the hospital, he can be accomodated.

Dr. Barken says before this procedure is undertaken, tests are made to assess the extent of the obstruction and to determine its precise location. At this point other tests are done to be sure there is no cancer present or any prostatic infection.

A catheter is left in the bladder until the following morning and then removed.

Dr. Lester A. Klein, an urologist at the Scripps Clinic in La Jolla, California says that at first the balloon treatment was effective on only about thirty percent of the cases. But now with doctors screening out the patients with poor chances for success with the balloon dilation, Dr. Klein says there is a success rate of eighty-six percent.

Dr. Klein is the designer of one of the balloon devices used in the operation and does the procedure himself at Scripps.

Dr. Barken has developed a similar technique using the same principles as Dr. Klein, but without the use of the sophisticated multiple balloons. This helps bring the cost down tremendously.

At this point in mid 1990, urologists who use the balloon technique have praise for it. They say it is effective, and is easy to do with the least amount of stress and worry on the patient. It is non-surgical, and as of yet, there have been no side effects reported. These three factors make it a favorite with patients as well especially when contrasted with surgery.

Another factor is the cost. While few hard figures are obtainable, one Boston urologist said the average total cost for a balloon dilation in the hospital is about $3,600. For the same TURP operation the cost is about $12,000. TURP surgery is one of the operations that remove part or all of the growth in the prostate.

A medical writer in the Wall Street Journal estimated that more than 2,000 of these balloon treatments have been done. A CBS news report about the same procedure said that over 5,000 of them have been undertaken in the past two years.

After three years of watching the balloon treatment, many researchers and doctors now find that the balloon dilation of the urethra is not long lasting enough to make it ultimately practical. If the balloon method of treatment for BPH interests you, be sure to ask for all available medical literature, medical tests, and information on patient responses to the procedure.

Not everyone agrees with the use of the balloon dilation treatment. Dr. John W. Schumacher, M.D. from Minneapolis says that this ignores the 10 percent of those who do get a TURP operation and the pathologist find that they have prostate cancer as well. Dr. Schumacher says that if a hundred thousand balloon treatments are used for BPH, then ten thousand of those men who have Stage A or B Cancer won't find out about it—perhaps until it's too late to cure them.

Dr. William J. Somers, M.D., a urologist, agrees. He puts hidden cancer of BPH patients at twenty to twenty-five percent.

He says that the use of the balloon dilation or drugs to reduce BPH symptoms is actually doing those twenty-five percent of the patients with hidden cancer a disservice. Other experts say these hidden cancers are rarely fatal in nature.

He maintains that there is no accurate way of determining who has prostate cancer and who doesn't. Biopsy and ultrasound can help, but he says unless shavings of the gland are examined in a pathology laboratory, the cancer can metastasize and no one will know about it until it's too late.

Dr. Walter Desmond, Jr. Ph.D. and research manager at Hybritech in San Diego has a slightly different view of the evaluation of the scrapings from a TURP operation. His firm makes a test called the PSA to evaluate the prostate specific antigen level in the blood. A high level can indicate the strong possibility of a silent cancer in the prostate.

He says that some pathologists fail to examine all of the tissue taken out during a TURP operation. Those who don't evaluate all of the scrapings are shortchanging the patient.

He says the odds are even greater that a hidden cancer may be missed because a proper TURP cuts out the central part of the prostate tissue. The great majority of small cancers start not at the center of the prostate but near or on the surface of the lobes of the prostate, and these areas are often never touched by the surgeon's electric knife when he cuts out the new canal for the urine to pass through.

Dr. Desmond seems to be saying that if pathologists are finding small cancers in the ten percent, or as high as 30 percent by some scientific evaluations of the TURP scrapings, then the true figure must be much higher than that taking into consideration the two factors presented here.

His slant seems to be that a chemical test such as PSA offers a much better method to detect early prostate cancer than any other method.

Laser Minor Surgery

Yes, the laser is now being used in a few of the estimated 400,000 operations in the United States each year to treat BPH, or the restriction of urine flow in the urethra through the prostate.

Dr. Israel Barken, a urologist in San Diego, writing in the *Cancer Communication* newsletter from PAACT, says that the increase in use of the laser is partly due to the recent development of a new type of laser fiber that can help the doctor to apply the laser energy in the tight space inside the prostate.

In the past, the laser's energy was aimed forward, in the longitudinal direction of the fiber. This made maneuvering the energy difficult in the small urethra area of the prostate. Now it is possible to direct the laser 90 degrees to the longitudinal axis of the fiber, making it easier to use the laser inside the prostate.

Tissue hit by the laser undergoes changes for five to six weeks. At the end of that time, a new cavity has been created and is lined by a new covering layer of cells. The dead tissue has been evacuated through the urine during those weeks, but without any problems to the patient.

This new laser approach to the prostate makes this procedure appealing to the patient, since recovery is quick and complications are negligible. Like any other medical procedure, the laser's use must stand the test of time.

General anesthesia may not be needed. The procedure takes only a few minutes to perform. There is no blood loss during the procedure or after the operation.

There is no risk of absorption of fluids during the operation. The whole operation can be performed in a doctor's office, eliminating the cost of hospitalization.

However, there are some disadvantages to laser use in the prostate: undertrained physicians may use the laser in such a way as to perforate the prostate toward the rectum, or they might injure the sphincter, causing incontinence. Too deep a penetration with the laser in the prostate could cause impotence.

The laser fibers are expensive, but avoidance of hospitalization helps reduce the overall cost to the patient. The big drawback is that when the laser is used to "clean out" the prostate, there is no tissue left to be analyzed in the lab for possible cancerous cells. With the TURP or the "rotor rooter" system, the extracted tissue is examined.

The choice whether or not to try laser surgery for advanced BPH is up to the patient and his urologist. The techniques and equipment in this field are bound to become more perfected and practical in the years to come.

Other Non Major Surgical Approaches

Ultrasound

Prostatic ultrasound diagnostic procedure is a very effective test. It projects an image of the whole prostate gland on a television screen. A videotape can be made of it for later evaluation and to use as a baseline for checking on the patient in subsequent years.

The front and the back of the prostate can be seen. Its size, weight, volume, and shape, as well as the internal structure, can be viewed and analyzed.

For the patient, ultrasound testing offers a safe, noninvasive test with no radiation and no wire cutting. It is short in duration and gives the patient little discomfort.

The ultrasound often can detect small lesions that would not be found during a routine rectal exam.

The ultrasound can be used after an increased PSA test result, in the viewing mode, to double-check for any cancer, and if it is found, to pinpoint the placement, size, type, and extent of the growth.

In the use of ultrasound in prostate treatment, the ultrasound waves attack the tissue blocking the prostate. The unwanted tissue is turned into a pulp and dislodged and sucked out of the body by an aspirator.

In the future, ultrasound may be used much more by doctors dealing with the prostate. This method offers several advantages to the physician and the patient.

Dr. Terrence R. Malloy, chief of urology at Pennsylvania Hospital in Philadelphia, attacks the enlarged prostate tissue with ultrasound waves. The tissue is turned into a pulp and dislodged and then sucked out of the body by an aspirator.

Some research is now being done with microwaves. They are aimed directly at the enlarged prostate. Testing is now underway to see what results are of attempts to shrink the enlarged prostate tissue, thereby relieving the pressure on the urethra.

Another experimental type of minor surgery is the use of cryogenics. This utilizes a probe through the penis and urethra and into the heart of the enlarged prostate. The probe then releases liquid nitrogen into the enlarged tissue.

This intensely cold fluid freezes and shrinks the tissue and destroys it which relieves the pressure on the urethra. More experiments and results of this type of cryosurgery will be reported in the first half of the 1990's we are sure.

Stents

Another device that is in experimental use and development is called a stent. This is a springlike spiral or sheath that physically holds the urethra open much as shoring on a tunnel keeps the walls from caving in.

Some devices are now on the market, and a lot of study is being done on them. From a layman's viewpoint, they look simple and foolproof, but they aren't.

They are strong enough to keep the prostate from putting pressure on the urethra and interfering with urine flow. Many of these devices are of tubular metal mesh and are self-anchoring once they're in place. There is no problem putting them in the right place, and it's done in about 20 minutes with a local anesthetic.

Medical experts say that the basic drawback to them is the problem of the body rejecting them as foreign objects. Infections occur and other problems develop. Work is continuing to find the perfect solution to the problems of the stents.

The Tulip Procedure

One of the newest procedures for relieving BPH pressures is called the TULIP. This stands for Transurethral Ultrasound-Guided Laser-Induced Prostatectomy. This combines a resectoscope tube with an inflatable balloon at the tip, an ultrasound probe, and a laser.

The ultrasound image sent back from the probe

helps the physician aim the laser more accurately. The laser beam shoots through the balloon and the urethra and heats the prostate tissue, burning away the unwanted sections. This tissue is later passed out of the body through the urine during the next five to eight weeks.

More work is being done on this procedure as well.

Transurethral Incision

Another method for treating some BPH problems is the transurethral incision of the prostate. This consists simply of one or two incisions that are made at the opening of the bladder into the prostate using an electrical knife or a laser. Such cuts allow the gland to split slightly to each side, which often relieves the pressure on the urethra and allows easier urination.

This method is especially good for men with small prostates and may provide the same results of the more complicated TURP operation and with less inconvenience and suffering for the patient.

In many cases, this solves the problem dramatically and restores urination to the pre-BPH levels.

Can Drugs Be Used Instead of Surgery?

Over the years there have been many attempts made to find a drug that would shrink the prostate gland. The scientists worked on the belief that the enlargement of the prostate had something to do with the male hormone production.

This led to the use of female hormones that did shrink the prostate and help the BPH problem and reduced or eliminated the symptoms. The only trouble was that it also reduced and eliminated the male sex drive and often led to sterilization and impotence of the patient.

After that the lab men worked on drugs that would simply block the production of testosterone produced in the testicles. They came up with Leuprolide (lupron) which blocks ninety percent of the body's total production.

Another companion drug used at the same time, Flutamide (eulexin), eliminates the other ten percent of testosterone made by the adrenal gland.

What these drugs do is effectively castrate the man by chemical action. This reduces the male libido, his sex drive, and sterilizes him and makes him impotent. These are mighty tough side effects even for a man in his seventies just to shrink the size of the prostate.

These drugs are most often chosen when a man has an extreme case of BPH or cancer of the prostate, and his sexual life is no longer a factor in his life whether he's 65 or 80 years.

For most men the sexual side of life is always a vital part of their existence. It's like watching a shiny new bus stop at your corner. It's nice to know the bus service is always there, even though you seldom use it any more.

Relaxation Drugs

Some urologists find that the use of a drug such as Minipress (prazosin hydrochloride) will relax the smooth muscles surrounding the prostate. The purpose here is to get these muscles to relax or loosen to allow the prostate to expand slightly outward and thereby ease the internal pressure on the urethra.

A second drug used for the same purpose of relaxation of the muscles around the prostate is Terazosin. It relaxes the muscles and greatly reduces the spasms that these muscles frequently have which slow or prevent urination.

BPH is a highly subjective ailment. What bothers one patient may be little more than a minor and unnoticed irritant to another. Some patients who use one of these drugs may report relief from some of their symptoms, while others say they have no effect whatsoever on their life style.

Tests have shown some urologists that the use of Minipress and Dibenzyline drugs have made specific improvement in patient symptoms. Studies have been done to measure the voiding flow rate and residual urine before and after the use of these drugs, with an average of 60% improvement.

Proscar

One of the new drugs on the market that can be used in conjunction with BPH is Proscar, from Merck & Co. It was approved by the FDA late in 1992 and went on sale at once.

Proscar is said to block an enzyme that stimulates prostate growth. Merck researchers say that the male hormone testosterone undergoes changes in the prostate gland, and this is believed to be the primary factor in unwanted prostate growth in men thirty years or older.

By blocking this enzyme and refusing to let it change the testosterone, it can stop the growth of the prostate.

Using 350 patients in one clinical test, Proscar reduced the size of enlarged prostates an average of 28 percent. One-third of the test patients also had "some improvement" in their urine flow.

Dr. John McConnell, assistant professor of urology at the University of Texas Southwestern Medical Center in Dallas, said: "Proscar is highly effective. It does shrink the prostate." He also said that since only one-third of the patients had an improvement in urine flow, Proscar is not applicable to all men nor to all BPH cases.

One good thing about Proscar is that it has minimal side effects. Studies show that 97 percent of patients using Proscar who were not impotent before using Proscar can maintain their ability to have erections.

One drawback is that Proscar takes three to six months of use before it shows any effect, and then the patient would need to take the drug for the rest of his life.

Another drawback is that the use of Proscar can lower the PSA level in some patients. This masking of the real PSA level could cover up the early beginnings of cancer that the PSA test would otherwise show.

If you take Proscar, be sure to have other cancer-checking tests such as the rectal digital exam and ultrasound at regular intervals to catch any developing cancer.

Many patients say they feel better and urinate better when they use Proscar. At this early point in the history of this drug, it is speculation to say whether this is the result of the drug or from a psychological boost because the patient thinks that the drug will help him.

Proscar is there as an alternative. If it interests you, talk to your doctor about it.

Hytrin . . . Available Now

There is one drug on the market now, and available, that researchers at Abbott Laboratories of Chicago say will do the job of relieving BPH symptoms.

This is Hytrin, Abbott's brand of terazosin, approved by the FDA in 1987 as a once-a-day pill for high blood pressure.

Dr. Atul Laddau, Abbott's head of clinical research, says their own clinical tests of two years show that Hytrin relieves pressure on the urethra almost immediately and reduces other symptoms in about two thirds of the test patients with BPH. Some urologists are using Hytrin because it is now on the market, and because of the reported quick results. You don't wait three months for relief here.

There are some unfortunate side effects with Hytrin. These are said to be dizziness, fatigue and occasionally fainting attacks. Even considering these side effects. Hytrin, with its two-thirds success rate and its availability, should be one of the drugs that you talk to your doctor about. There are other terazosin medications on the market beside Hytrin. Cost of these pills is said to be about $15 to $20 a month.

Up to two years ago there had been a thriving over the counter and through the mails business of selling non-prescription compounds and "cures" and treatments for BPH.

Several years ago the Post Office Department began challenging many of these products sold through the mail on grounds that they were advertised misleadingly, and that they did not do what they claimed to do. Simple misrepresentation which could ban them from the mail.

That campaign by the U.S. postal authorities put a lot of people out of business who were selling various mail order non-prescription products to treat the prostate.

In March of 1990, the Food and Drug Adminstration said it would ban the sale of *all non-prescription drugs* used to treat enlargement of the prostate gland. The FDA said their review of the products found little evidence that any of them eliminated, arrested or treated the condition called benign prostatic hypertrophy. There was no date given for enforcing the ban or activating it.

The FDA, evidently not keeping up with current developments in the field, said surgery was the only effective treatment for BPH. A lot of urologists and specialists in the drug field will argue long and hard with their dictum with the various minor-surgical techniques we've discussed so far and the new drugs being developed.

What the FDA order does is ban non-prescription products that are *advertised* for the treatment of the prostate. They did not, and can not ban the sale of certain chemicals or compounds that have been considered by many since the Feinblatt/Gant study in 1958, to be beneficial to reduce BPH symptoms. These chemicals, mainly amino acids, are used in many of the soon to be banned products.

The study was conducted by Dr. Henry M. Feinblatt and Dr. Julian C. Gant and reported in the Journal of the Maine Medical Association in March of 1958, Volume 49, Number 3.

The study deals with the "Value of glycine, alanine and glutamic acid combination," in the treatment of BPH.

These three chemicals have generally been used by dozens, perhaps hundreds of non-prescription compounds aimed at the general public since 1958.

Were these remedies straight out of the Wild West's Medicine Man's wagon of hokum, or do they have some beneficial results that the traditionalist medical men on the FDA panels refuse to recognize?

Let's look at the Feinblatt/Gant study that started it all.

The doctors had been using these three amino acids to treat their allergy patients. One of the patients mentioned that his urinary problems had improved since he'd been taking the medications from the doctors.

This stirred their imagination and the two medical men decided to try the three way amino acid combination on a group of non-allergy patients. The tests proved that these BPH sufferers had a dramatic relief from their urinary and BPH symptoms.

They moved from there to a clinically stringent test. A group of 40 patients with benign prostatic hyperplasia was treated with glycine-alanine-glutamic acid capsules for three months.

The patient age range was from 37 to 75 years and weigh from 101 to 192 pounds. BPH complaints ranged in duration at the start of the test from one to six years by various patients.

Placebo capsules were given to half of the patients and the amino acids to half. The patients response results over three months were charted. (Understand here that most such tests should be conducted over six months for best reliability.)

Results of the clinical tests were published in this way. For the control group taking the amino acids, the doctors said the size of the prostate was reduced in 92% of the cases. Nocturia was relieved in 95% of cases. Urgent urination was relieved in 81% and frequency in 73%. Discomfort was reduced in 71% of the cases. No such results were observed in the placebo taking control patients.

Other medical authorities have conducted tests along the same lines to confirm or deny the Feinblatt/Gant findings.

In the Journal of the American Geriatrics Society in 1962, Dr. Frederick Damrau of New York City reported such a test. His conclusions were similar. He said the combination of the three amino acids were used in a controlled crossover test in forty cases of BPH. After three months on the test the patients reported nocturia was relieved or reduced in 95% of cases, urgency down in 81%, frequency lowered in 73% and delayed urination in 70%. Dr. Damrau said there were no adverse side effects or adverse reactions to the amino acids.

Other evidence the FDA ignored or discounted comes from Japan where a series of nine clinical tests were conducted at the department of urology of Kyoto University in Kyoto.

Some of these tests were double blind, which means there was no way the participants could have any idea if they were receiving the test material or a placebo.

The tests were published in the *Acta Urological Japonica,* volume 14, 1968.

Results for the amino acids therapy for hypertrophy of the prostate showed that the glycine-alanine-glutamic acid capsules were administered to thirty six cases of diagnosed uncomplicated BPH. The capsules gave satisfactory results in relieving subjective and objective symptoms and no side effects were observed in any of the patients.

In another of the tests, statistical results showed that improvement of symptoms were as follows:

- Urinary frequency reduced in 77.7%
- Nocturia relieved in 68.4%. Difficulty of urination relieved 77.3%
- Feeling of residual urine relieved in 71.4%

Side effects were found in only one case and that was relieved with a gastrointestinal drug.

Now, one of the obvious questions is this: If these amino acids are so good, as these tests tend to show, why hasn't one of the huge pharmaceutical giants leaped on the band wagon and brought out a tested, recognized and approved by FDA combination of these amino acids for the prostate sufferers?

The logical answer could be that their own testing did not match the results of the tests shown above. Or, the situation may be that the amino acids would not be a "proprietary" compound that they could patent, protect and profit from. It would be similar to spending millions to test a salt pill, and bring it out only to find that every other company could make the same salt pill.

Over the Counter

Just what does the March, 1990 publicity release by the FDA mean? Will there still be over the counter preparations designed to help with BPH problems by the end of the year, or into 1994? Only the FDA knows.

A check of health food and nutrition specialty stores in mid 1993 showed at least five products on the market. Many of these tend to be regional and there well could be twenty or fifty more out there. These are shown as examples of what's on the market now. We do not judge any of them but present them here as another element of the BPH real-life picture for the layman.

Prostate Plus

This product came to our attention through a multi-page tabloid type newspaper mailed to a name and address (or current occupant). It was a national mass mailing and held a 3/4 page story and advertisement for Prostate Plus.

Prostate Plus was described as a "Total nutritional support for a healthy prostate." It went on to say that it: "provides every nutrient known to benefit a healthy, well-functioning prostate gland." Since it is advertised as a nutritional supplement and not a medical treatment, perhaps it will get around the FDA broadsword.

What's in it? l-Glycine, l-Alanine, l-glutamic acid, zinc, raw prostate, saw palmetto, pumpkin seed concentrate, vitamin E, golden rod, and flaxseed oil.

Ninety capsules cost you $14.95 in the store.

Prostone

Prostone comes from the Enzymatic Therapy people in Green Bay, Wisconsin. The Prostone No. 190 is described this way: "The nutrients in this formula including zinc, Vitamin A, essential fatty acids and amino acids, are vital for proper prostate function."

What's in it? Oil concentrate from wheat germ and safflower seeds, linoleic acid from safflower seed oil, intrinsic glandular lipids, lecithin, L-Glutamic acid, L-Alanine, Amenoacetic acid, Prostate tissue, Vitamin B6, Vitamin A from fish liver oil, Zinc chelate, bee pollen and saw palmetto berries extract.

Sixty capsules will cost you $11.95.

Raw Prostate With Gaba

This product is made up exclusively of raw bovine prostate and gamma amino butyric acid. That's about all we know about it except that it comes from Country Life, a large maker of health food additives and products. It's on the market. Glad they told us it was bovine prostate. Ninety tablets will cost you $13.00

Prostatrophic Concentrate

This one is made up entirely from raw bovine prostate. One such ingredient indicated it had been freeze dried. Here 100 tablets are priced at $8.00.

Search

This small bottle of sixty tablets was priced at $10 and the ingredients were listed as raw bovine prostate.

So, we've talked about the non-surgical, minor surgery and drug type of treatments for BPH. Where do we go from here? If none of the other methods are right for you, your urologist may suggest traditional surgery for your BPH. What's that? Move right on to the next chapter and find out.

5

Traditional Prostate Surgery

When you and your urologist decide that the best way to handle your BPH or other prostate trouble is surgery, you have another decision to make. Which type of surgery will do the job that needs to be done?

Today, about 95% of all BPH surgery uses the standard transurethral resection of the prostate, or TURP, as it is called.

Your urologist will explain to you in detail what this surgery involves.

The TURP is what surgeons call a closed operation. That simply means that there is no incision made in the body to get at the problem.

The TURP uses a surgical instrument that is inserted into the penis through the urethra. He'll point out to you that this is done after the use of anesthesia. The instrument is a nonflexible hollow tube that extends into the narrowed portion of the urethra inside the prostate.

Inside this tube the urologist will insert a fiber optic micro-lens system that doctors call a resectoscope. This device includes a fiber optics light source, a lens and an electric wire element for surgery. The light inside the urethra lets the doctor see the problem and determine the severity of the problem.

The electrical wire loop emerges from the end of the tube and is used to cut away the prostatic tissue. Power is applied to the electric loop by the use of a foot switch when the surgeon wants to cut.

As he does this, the surgeon is watching the procedure through a lens that is located just outside the end of the penis.

When bleeding occurs inside the urethra, another foot pedal is pressed and the bleeding part is sealed off by cauterization. During the surgery the entire area is washed by glycine.

After the surgeon decides that he has removed enough of the enlarged prostate, the chips and shavings of the prostate tissue are removed with the glycine wash and sent to a pathologist who studies them to see if there are any beginnings of cancer of the prostate.

The surgeon may elect to remove most or all of the prostate but he will not harm the prostate's surgical capsule. This new hole that has been created through the overgrown prostate now becomes a urinary canal. This means that the prostate enlargement tissue was growing around the urethra gradually closing it down and narrowing it. The inner walls of the urethra have been cut away carving a new canal through the prostatic tissue growth.

After the cutting is done, a thin, flexible rubber or plastic tube is then passed through the penis and urethua and into the bladder so urine can be drawn from the bladder.

This tube remains in place for a few days because of

some bleeding that may take place in the prostate. When the tube is removed, the patient will be able to urinate normally again.

This catheter, used after the TURP surgery, consists of three lumens or tubes. One is used to send in and remove a wash of saline solution, salt water, into the bladder to irrigate and clean it. This saline solution usually is used for twenty-four hours after surgery.

The second tube is used to draw off urine. The third usually has a small balloon attached and is inflated so the catheter will not fall out.

The catheter to draw urine from the bladder stays in place for two days after surgery.

Most patients feel good enough to get out of bed a day after surgery and are feeling much better after four days. Yes, you can walk and talk and sit down with the catheter in place. It usually comes out on the second day and no pain is involved.

The surgeon will deflate the balloon and the catheter can then simply slide out. The following day, most patients are discharged and sent home. Hospital stay: two days.

Most TURP patients get a prescription for antibiotics to be taken by mouth for one to two weeks after the surgery. This is a precaution to ward off any infection.

Post surgical suggestions from his urologists will probably advise the patient to take hot baths rather than showers for a while, drink lots of fluids, avoid spicy foods and watch out not to become constipated.

There won't be any touch football games for a while, but most of the patient's activities can be resumed, including driving, sitting at a desk and taking walks.

If there is any trouble it probably will be a slight

burning during the first two weeks when he urinates, and even small amounts of blood in his urine. If this happens, the patient should call his urologist and report the problem just to be on the safe side.

When can you get back to work? These are general guidelines. You'll follow your doctor's orders here. They will depend on the doctor, the patient and how well he recovers. Generally: If you do heavy manual labor, best to wait four to six weeks. Moderate labor will call for three to four weeks of vacation. The mental giant behind a desk or in a white collar position can get back in his harness after two weeks.

One caution. The TURP patient should hold off any sexual activity for six weeks after surgery. This will allow the canal through the prostate to heal completely.

The TURP surgery is performed about 400,000 times a year in the U.S. and the numbers probably are rising with the increase in percentage of our male population reaching the BPH age.

Dangers and Side Effects

Let's take a closer look at TURP and the statistical dangers and side effects.

1. Retrograde Ejaculation. This is in effect defacto sterilization. There is no other way to describe it. A vital part of the reproductive system in the male is contained in the prostate and other elements are injected into and flow through the urethra situated inside the prostate.

When most or all of the prostate is removed, the fluid that the prostate produces to lubricate and carry the sperm down the urethra is also gone. Now when orgasm takes place, muscular contractions propel the spermatozoa and fluid from the prostate and seminal vesicles into the prostatic urethra.

At the same time this happens, the neck of the bladder closes so the fluids must go down the urethra and out the penis. But after TURP surgery, this bladder neck closure is usually cut away to provide more space for the urine flow.

With the bladder neck open, the sperm and the fluid take the path of least resistance and are propelled into the bladder instead of out the penis.

This is called retrograde ejaculation. The sensation of the orgasm is the same for the man, there just isn't any outside ejaculation.

With many TURP patients this is not a problem. Most men in the good TURP surgery candidate pool are no longer interested in fathering children. In most of the cases when a patient is told about this drawback and result of the TURP, he will not have any major problems with it. The trouble comes when a patient is not told about retrograde ejaculation and finds out on his own and is furious that he wasn't informed before the operation.

In the extreme case where fatherhood is still desired, the ejaculate can be retrieved after the next urination after the orgasm, and the semen gathered and preserved and used in an insertion procedure into the woman's vagina, the same as any artificial insemination. It works.

2. Bleeding. TURP involves a lot of cutting of tissue and the enclosed blood vessels. Bleeding is a natural course of events. Most of the bleeding is stopped during the operation by cauterization.

As with any cut or wound, a scab develops. This

should stay for two or three weeks and then fall off. By then the blood vessel should be healed. If the scab falls off sooner bleeding usually begins and shows up in the urine.

This happens in only about one percent of all TURP patients and is often caused by straining to pass a stool. Usually this bleeding can be helped by a patient drinking lots of fluids to cleanse the area. Only rarely is there a need for the patient to be readmitted to the hospital to correct the condition.

3. *Incontinence.* (The inability to control voiding of urine.) This is one of the big fears of a TURP surgical patient. It is embarrassing and distressing, and can lead a patient to total social isolation.

Incontinence happens to from one to four percent of all TURP patients. Many urologists claim it is less frequent, and say it can be the result of the normal surgical risk factor.

The problem comes when the electric knife cuts too near the sphincter voluntary muscles which control the flow of urine. If these muscles are damaged then the patient may become incontinent.

The other means of continence is the external urethral sphincter. Damage here can lead to a stress type of incontinence.

Incontinence after a TURP operation does not have to be permanent or irreversible. There are drugs that can be used to relieve the situation. Another possibility here is the use of an artificial sphincter.

At any rate this is one of the areas that you should discuss with your doctor prior to any prostate operation.

4. *Impotency.* Experts in this field say about five per-

cent of all TURP patients come out of the operation and are impotent even though they were not that way going in.

Impotency is simply a man's inability to achieve an erection, or to maintain it long enough for vaginal penetration.

The "manliness" of a male is a highly subjective area, and statistics on this element may be dramatically wrong in either direction. Many men may say they are able to achieve an erection and have intercourse when they are 70, 75, even 80. But age and other problems may have reduced that libido drastically so that even they were not totally cognizant of their ability to achieve a working erection. Time and age does this to all men.

Sometimes such an operation is a handy whipping boy for the sudden realization of impotency.

In any case, impotency is a fact of life for some of the men who have TURP operations, and you should know about it now. There is one sure way to develop impotency in a TURP patient. That is to damage one or both of the nerve bundles that are on each side of the prostate. These bundles are outside of the true capsule of the prostate. That means they are well outside of the area a surgeon's electric knife should be operating to remove the prostatic tissue clogging the urethra. This is to say that a TURP properly carried out, should not harm these nerve bundles and that should not be the reasons for any impotency.

Some psychologists say that sex is at least 75% mental. This is why the cause of impotency, especially in men from 60 to 90 is extremely difficult to tie down. It may have been there before the operation and not recognized. The operation might create a psychological block preventing the erection. A now and then lack of a man's ability to "get it up" is not uncommon even in younger men. The trauma of the operation, even the thought of some danger to a patient's "manhood" and a negative spousal situation all can combine to create a psychosomatic impotency. This may be of a short or long duration.

There are drugs that can be used to help this impotency, and several devices that will be covered in a later chapter. Impotency, while not a large factor, is one that the surgery candidate for TURP should be well aware of.

TUIP: Trans Urethral Incision Prostate

The TUIP is simply a pair of incisions made on the sides of the bladder neck that closes the bladder off from the urethra. The incisions are made through the urethra and is a simple procedure. Urologists are not sure why this works for the relief of BPH problems, but it does. Often urine peak flow is greatly increased, getting up at night is reduced and hesitation and some of the other less serious BPH problems are lessened.

This procedure is much like a TURP for the equipment used and the insertion. The electric knife makes only the two incisions and no removal of prostatic tissue is done. This is another option a patient with really bothersome BPH has to find relief.

The Suprapubic Prostatectomy

In this surgery an incision is made below the navel and to a point just above the pubis. An alternative may be an incision just above the pubic hair. The incisions will be from four to six inches long.

The surgeon goes in here cutting through skin and its lining. The patient's muscles covering the bladder are carefully separated and the sac covering the abdominal wall is pulled back. Then an incision is made in the bladder.

Now the surgeon removes the prostate gland and the tissue is examined for any evidence of cancer. Cauterization or sutures close off all bleeding vessels. The stitches will dissolve later.

When bleeding is controlled, the surgeon inserts a catheter in the penis and up through the urethra into the bladder to irrigate it. The bladder is then emptied.

Now a second catheter is inserted directly into the bladder. It will leave the body just below the navel. This catheter is used to drain urine and irrigation fluids from the bladder after the operation. It is larger than the one in the penis and more effective.

Continuous irrigation of the bladder and the prostate area is continued for two days. The large catheter is removed in a day or two but the penile catheter is left in for six or seven days. This allows urine to be removed from the bladder and lets the prostate area heal.

After the catheter is removed the patient usually can urinate normally.

Retropubic Prostatectomy

In this surgery the same type incision is made as in the suprapubic operation. The muscle is separated and the sac containing the intestines is moved away from the bladder.

Now the surgeon makes an incision into the prostate capsule and removes the enlarged gland. The tissue removed is tested by a pathologist to determine if there is any cancerous growths present.

Now the surgeon sutures or cauterizes the bleeding vessels and the catheter with the three way tube is placed into the bladder. This catheter is usually the same type as used in a TURP operation. Next the balloon is inflated to keep the catheter in place.

All that is left is for the surgeon to "close." The prostate capsule is sutured shut and the muscles, fascia and skin are put back in place and stitched closed.

This operation differs from the previous one since the bladder itself was not opened. It's slightly simpler with less violation of the body. This means there is no need for the second catheter through the belly to drain the bladder.

The draining and irrigation of the prostate needed can be done with the usual three-way catheter. Most urologists say that this operation is less stressful to the patient since the bladder is not cut open, so it doesn't have to recover.

General recovery procedures and time is about the same for either type of operation. Which type your urologist might suggest would be determined by the individual patient's condition and sometimes the doctor's preference.

In surgery for the prostate, the general rule is that a medium sized enlarged prostate and smaller ones can be successfully removed by the TURP method. However when the gland swells in size to over fifty to sixty grams, the urologist will usually do one of the other operations because of the difficulty in scraping out that much tissue and drawing it out of the urethra.

In these cases the larger prostate removal by the retropubic or suprapubic is simply the most efficient method to be used for the well being of the patient.

Other Types Of Prostate Surgery

Perineal prostatectomy is another kind of open surgery for the prostate but it is seldom used today. This procedure is quick and simple to do, but almost always severs the nerve bundles that control erection and leaves the patient impotent.

Doctors back in the 1930's often used a two stage operation for the prostate. The first stage was opening and draining the bladder. Then two weeks later they would go in and remove the prostate. It is seldom used today.

With the new treatments now coming into focus for the prostate, particularly BPH, there may be a general slowing in the number of surgeries needed. Any surgery has risks but with the prostate the risks seem to be reasonable in regards to impotence and incontinence, the two problems most men fear the most.

With the development of the new drugs, we may see products that will cause the enlarged prostate to shrink without objectionable side effects. With the increased use of the balloon as at least a temporary treatment for BPH, and other inventive methods, some experts are predicting that the use of surgery will not be required as often in future years as it is today. Only time will tell. As the public learns more about the male prostate and BPH, more men will demand non-intrusive treatments whenever possible. Right now a lot of men are hanging their hopes on the new drugs Hytrin and Proscar.

6

Infectious And Noninfectious Prostatitis

Prostatitis is an inflammation of the prostate gland and it is one of the most common of men's diseases. There is no age limit here—prostatitis attacks any man from teenager to grandfather in his nineties.

How do you know if you have it? You'll be absolutely certain that something is wrong. Prostatitis is not subtle. A case of acute prostatitis may bring on a sudden fever, chills, nausea and vomiting besides urgency of urination, hesitancy, burning pain during urination and even pus or blood in the urine.

Most family physicians who diagnose acute prostatitis will suggest the patient go to a specialist, the urologist.

Prostatitis can be caused by infection, irritation and congestion or a combination of these problems. Many urologists will tell you that sometimes there is no apparent cause of the condition.

This ailment does respond well to treatment, even if it is a bit slow sometimes.

The infectious type of prostatitis results from some microorganism or bacteria that has invaded the prostate. With its tough outer shell, the prostate is hard to get into. But it can be infected through the bloodstream, the lymph system, and the urine.

A lot of the infections come from bacteria from the colon. However, antibiotics now can be used to knock out this type of infection before it gets serious.

Bacteria can get into the prostate from sexual contact. The yeast infections as well as gonorrhea can be sexually transmitted. This danger is just another reason to be safe in your sexual life, wear a condom.

Some people can develop prostatitis simply by eating or drinking certain foods or beverages. On the avoidance list for some people are coffee, gin, red wine and Scotch whiskey. Aromatic oils are used to flavor these drinks and that is what irritates the prostate and sets it to complaining.

We mentioned gonorrhea as one problem. At one time it was the most prevalent infection of the male urogenital tract. But now with the better antibiotics, this sexually transmitted social disease can usually be cured quickly. A fast cure has the added benefit of stopping the infection before it can travel to the prostate.

Sometimes abscesses do develop in the prostate from gonorrhea. This is often because the man has an antibiotic resistant strain or did not get prompt enough treatment to kill off the disease quickly. The abscesses result in the same usual symptoms of acute prostatitis.

A urine sample usually shows up minute amounts of the prostate emissions and microscopic examination of the emissions will help the doctor determine what bacteria have made their attack and that will determine what treatment is prescribed. Most prostatitis clears up quickly with the proper medication.

Chronic Prostatitis

Sometimes the condition will be cleared up, or seem to be back to normal, only to have it flare up again. Cases like this are called chronic prostatitis.

At least this time the patient knows what he has and can get to the doctor quickly for early medication. If the drug used before didn't completely kill off the bacteria causing the problem, there is little chance the same medication will do any better during the next attack. Doctors watch for newly developed medications they hope will solve the problem. But so far there is no drug that will completely eliminate the chronic prostatitis problem.

Some urologists maintain that regular prostatic massage is one effective treatment for chronic prostatitis. Other urologists never use the massage treatment. Some urologists suggest masturbation if sex with a partner is not available. Almost all urologists will agree that the best way to empty the prostate of fluid is regular sexual activity of any type leading to ejaculation.

As with many of the ailments of the prostate, the old favorite treatment of the sitz bath, simply a hot tub bath, is well received by prostatitis sufferers. The heat from the water increases the circulation in the underwater area and that can help a number of problems.

Chronic prostatitis is not a good candidate problem to be corrected with surgery. It would be a case of overkill, like throwing out the baby with the bath water.

Urologists say that even if surgery were performed, the inflammation and pain could still come back in the prostatic capsule itself, even after most of the prostate had been removed. A prostatectomy also can bring up a whole new set of problems that the patient didn't have before.

Noninfectious Prostatitis

When a man gets serious pains and the urologist rules out infectious prostatitis, there has to be another cause. This might be from a whole group of problems and the doctors call this malady, noninfectious prostatitis.

The symptoms usually include lower-back pain, burning during urination, pain or slight discomfort after ejaculation, pelvic discomfort, and sometimes a slight but obvious bleeding during ejaculation.

The urologist will check the patient's prostate and often he'll find it to be filled with prostatic fluid, boggy and soft. It may or may not be enlarged and may or may not have any hard lumps or nodules.

For this problem, there are few simple answers, no easy solutions and no absolutes. The medical experts say that this noninfectious prostatitis could be caused by some kind of bug we can't see or don't know about yet, or it could be some form of inflammation that isn't infectious.

One constant seems to be that a prostatic massage will cause the patient to expel a great deal of prostatic fluid through the urethra and the penis. This often brings immediate relief to the patient.

Urologists aren't exactly sure why this works. They say that most men with normal prostates secrete a small amount of prostatic fluid every day. Most of this is passed off through the urine without the man being aware of it.

Upon sexual arousal this secretion can increase ten fold to do its job of helping to carry the sperm cells out the urethra and from the penis upon sexual climax.

When a man becomes aroused, and then frustrated and there is no orgasm, all of that extra prostatic fluid remains in the prostate. If this happens occasionally, the fluid is soon discharged a little at a time through the urine. But repeated frustrations after arousal, can mean a large buildup in the prostate and this will soon lead to some of the symptoms described above.

There are cases where a man can produce more prostatic fluid than he normally ejaculates during an orgasm. This again will create a buildup of the fluid and can result in problems. What this is saying is that there can be prostatic problems that have a direct relationship with a man's sex life, and this includes too little as well as too much sex.

There are cases where there are symptoms of prostatitis, but absolutely none of the usual causes are present. Some urologists feel that such a problem can come about entirely from stress. Some doctors say that there may be a lack of tone in some of the perineal muscles and this could result in the buildup of prostatic fluid. Nobody knows for sure.

This leads into the suggestion that there could be psychological reasons why some of these cases of prostatitis develop when there is none of the usual physical causes. Anxiety or stressful tensions dealing with sex, a man's job, his spouse, school or family—about almost anything, are now thought to be sufficient in some men to create symptoms of prostatitis even without any of the usual physical causes.

In some cases antibiotics seem to be helpful, even though there is no known bacteriological cause. Urologists are always aware of the placebo factor, especially in cases like these that may be partly stress or psychologically based.

Simply giving a man a pill and telling him that this will help his condition, often will help his condition. This is what doctors mean by the placebo effect. Placebos have traditionally been sugar pills with absolutely no curative powers whatsoever. However when a doctor gives the placebos to a patient and assures him that this should cure his problem after ten days, it often works.

This merges into the psychological and the psychosomatic aspects of healing, and in this area no one is right or wrong. What works, works, there is no reason to question it. Doctors and urologists say that the placebo effect must never be underestimated.

They point out in double blind clinical tests, the patients who are given the placebos without knowing it, often show a strong rate of improvement. The sugar pill certainly didn't do it, the placebo effect did. The patient thought he would get better, and somehow, he did get better.

In the chapter on case histories, we'll show several actual cases of both infectious and noninfectious prostatitis, and how the problems were resolved.

7

Prostate Cancer

Cancer is the word that has brought agonizing pain and terror to the last half of the twentieth century. To most people cancer means death. Many still think that a man with cancer has a death sentence. Not true.

Increasingly in this last decade of the century it is proving not necessarily so. There are hundreds of different kinds and types of cancers, the medical experts tell us, and some can and are being cured.

One of those types of cancer strikes men in their prostate. Cancer is described as being an uncontrolled growth of abnormal cells. Cancer cells can spread quickly throughout the body through the bloodstream and the lymph system. Wherever they live they create new tumors that begin replacing the normal tissue.

Some types don't move at all, some are aggressive and attack different parts of the body quickly. Cancer can develop in the lymphatic system, in bones, a man's lungs, chest, throat, colon, stomach, even his brain.

One of the areas cancer hits in a man is his prostate. When cancer strikes a man's prostate it is usually what doctors call a primary cancer. This simply means the cancer begins, originates, in the prostate and has not been transported there from some other cancer in another part of the body.

What Causes Prostate Cancer?

Scientists say there are hundreds of different kinds of cancer and they undoubtedly are caused by hundreds of different inciters. A few of the cancers have been researched enough so the medical people have the beginnings of the causes of them and can then go ahead and utilize some kind of antibody to stop or kill the cancer. Massive research is going on for many forms of cancer, but less than one percent of that work is being done on prostate cancer.

What this says is that there probably won't be a miracle cure for prostate cancer within the lifetimes of most of us. That, like some of the preventive inoculation vaccines we have, will have to be applied to our children or our grandchildren. So who can develop prostate cancer?

Unlike smoking and lung cancer, there isn't even a hint of what might cause prostate cancer. Most researchers have ruled out any of the usual work and behavior activities such as alcohol, diet, work place, smoking, venereal diseases, too much sex or too little, or any other currently defined lifestyle.

There is one exception: men who work in nearly constant exhaust fumes from cars and those exposed to cadmium in the wokr place, are found to be at slightly higher risks of prostate cancer than the rest of us.

The one constant in prostate cancer and man seems to be age. As with the enlargement of the prostate, cancer seems to strike older men. Yes, some men die of prostate cancer in their forties, but most of the confrontations with the disease comes when men are over sixty.

One researcher reports that the average age of men who are diagnosed as having cancer is seventy-two. Slightly over eighty percent of all prostate cancers reported come in men who are over the age of sixty-five.

Most doctors understand that by the age of eighty, nearly eighty percent of men have cancer of the prostate to some degree. It may have been dormant for years, or it may just be starting and of a type that will grow slowly. Most of these men will never develop any symptoms of prostate cancer and will die of some cause not related to their prostate cancer.

Most of our readers probably know someone who either has prostate cancer or has died of it. The American Cancer Society says that one out of eleven white Americans will develop cancer of the prostate during his lifetime. With black American men the figure is one in nine.

Nearly 100,000 prostate cancer cases are reported by doctors each year. With men living longer now each year, there is expected to be an increasing number of prostate cancers. Men are simply living longer now and that's when the disease develops.

The American Cancer Society reports that nearly 28,000 men died of prostate cancer last year.

What Can the Average Man Do?

The problem is far from hopeless. The key to any cancer, and especially prostate cancer, is to catch the problem as early as possible. Some urologists suggest that all men over forty should have a digital rectal examination once a year.

Most of these examinations will be negative, which is good news to the man examined. We do dozens of examinations each year on people and expect negative results. Cholesterol testing is done routinely on people in their twenties and thirties, but the problem usually isn't critical until much later in life. Chest X-rays are done routinely with usually a 99% negative result.

Testing for prostate cancer should be as routine for all men over forty. Yes, it's a bit uncomfortable, but not painful. It takes about three minutes in a doctor's office. Some urologists say the digital exam of the upper two lobes of the prostate will reveal ninety percent of prostate cancer. Other urologists think this is a bit high, but the exam should be made.

If such exams could catch 50% of starting prostate cancers in an early stage, most of those could be cured completely.

The big problem with prostate cancer is that it is a silent killer. It can show no symptoms at first. By the time it starts hurting, the cancer usually has spread into other parts of the body and it's often a matter of time until it kills the patient.

Scare Tactics?

Yes. Absolutely. If your reading this book does nothing more than makes you decide to have a yearly physical examination including a digital rectal exam of the prostate, that will be reward enough.

You could be saving your life with a digital examination by discovering a cancer early enough to cure it.

Right now, about sixty-four percent of prostate cancers are discovered while they are small. Of these men, almost eighty-four percent are still alive five years after their surgery. Doctors compile statistics on cancer patients and most consider a man cured after a 15 year free period. The secret is catching it early so all of the cancerous tissue can be removed so it can't spread or grow again. Ann Landers in her syndicated column has repeatedly pushed for greater awareness of testing to catch early cancer development. In one recent column she urged women to do the job this way. Whenever they go in for a mammogram, usually once a year, they should make an appointment for their husband to have his prostate checked by a digital exam or by the more expensive ultrasound probe. She urges women to do this so they won't become premature widows. The lady has a good idea.

The American Cancer Society reports that currently seventy-one percent of all patients with cancer of the prostate live for five years or more after treatment. That's for all cases whether diagnosed early or late.

The later the diagnosis, the worse the chance for a cure.

How Does Your Doctor Know It's Cancer?

More and more these days there is a push to try to catch prostate cancer in its earliest stages. This is a difficult job because very small cancers in the prostate traditionally have been from hard to impossible to detect by the traditional digital exam.

Now there are new tools to use to find these cancers. One of the best may be a simple blood test called the

PSA. That stands for Prostate Specific Antigen. Prostate antigen is a protein found only in the prostate tissue. It has long been known that when the prostate is cancerous, the antigen level is elevated. The problem has been in finding how much this elevation may be made when the cancers are small and can't be felt digitally.

Now with the PSA there has been enough research to make some general pointings.

Dr. William H. Cooner, of the Mobile Urology Group, P.A. and the Section of Urology, Springhill Memorial Hospital in Mobile, Alabama, reports several findings in the Alabama Medicine journal of the state medical association.

He points out that PSA levels reflect the volume of prostate tissue in the body, either benign or malignant, so will usually be elevated in the presence of BPH.

He shows a table of a test conducted by Hybritech Inc. of San Diego, correlating the PSA levels in 352 men with BPH and 533 men with proven prostate cancer.

The tests showed that in the BPH men when the level of antigen had risen to 4 units, BPH was likely by a ratio of 4 to 1. But when the antigen level lifted to 10 or more units, the likelihood of cancer was more likely by a ratio of 33 to 1.

Dr. Cooner also suggests the use of prostate ultrasonography as another diagnostic tool for screening patients who fall in the over 50 year category. This is done with a probe in the rectum and the use of ultrasound to reveal the tissue and mass in the prostate area.

Dr. Cooner concludes in his paper that we need to employ these two tools in a try to improve the ability to find curable cancers before they cause pain. He suggests that all men over 50 years should have a digital rectal elimination, then a PSA blood test, and a prostate ultrasound sonogram done as a baseline for future comparisons.

In a study at Johns Hopkins University School of Medicine, in Baltimore, Dr. Daniel Chan reports another PSA study. He says that on tested men at a level of 2.8 units of antigen there was considerable positive cancer results. He said that at 8.0 units there was a 94% chance of cancer, and when the PSA level reached 20.0 all of the patients had prostatic cancer.

At this time PSA looks like a tool that the urologists need to make more use of. What if it only catches two or three percent of early cancer cases. Those men, cured of their cancer, are going to be wildly enthusiastic about the benefits of the test.

As a parallel, how many positive readings do physical exams get these days from a routine chest X-ray? A dramatically low percentage.

What's the Diagnostic Sequence?

A patient goes to a urologist for many reasons. More and more family physicians are doing rectal digital examinations and when they find a lump or nodule on the prostate refer the patient to a specialist.

The urologist will confirm the digital diagnosis and then begin other tests to confirm or deny the first decision. He might do a biopsy of the prostate to test the tissue in the hard nodule. He almost certainly will do an ultrasound test and look at the findings on a sonogram or on a screen. There are also two blood tests he'll do for further confirmation of a cancerous growth.

As we pointed out before, there is no connection between an enlarged prostate and cancer. Usually the cancer does not press in on the urethra so there are none of the usual BPH symptoms which might get a man to go see his doctor.

There could be some symptoms a man might feel such as pain in the upper thighs, the pelvis or lower back, serious weight loss and shortness of breath. Symptoms such as these might mean nothing unusual, or be a sign of some other physical problem or disease—or they could be from cancer.

If the pain is related to prostate cancer, it may be a sign that the disease has spread outside of the prostate, and often it is too late to save the patient. That's why prostate cancer is often called a silent killer and the reason that preventive medicine must be practiced, the digital rectal exam, once a year.

Now, back to those tests to determine if the lump or nodule is cancer of the prostate. The drawing on the following page shows one way that cancer might grow in the prostate. This is viewed from the two lobes of the prostate that can be digitally examined.

A biopsy is the use of a needle inserted through the perineum or the rectum to remove a sample of tissue from the suspected nodule. This can be done by feel by the urologist or with the help of ultrasound to locate the specific area.

A biopsy can be done in the doctor's office or as an outpatient at a hospital and requires a local anesthesia. A relatively new way to take a biopsy is with what is called a "biopsy gun." It isn't a real gun. It's a biopsy needle that is used through the rectum and guided by ultrasound, but is "fired" in and out so quickly that the patient feels pressure and hears the sound the device makes, but he feels almost no pain. No anesthesia is given.

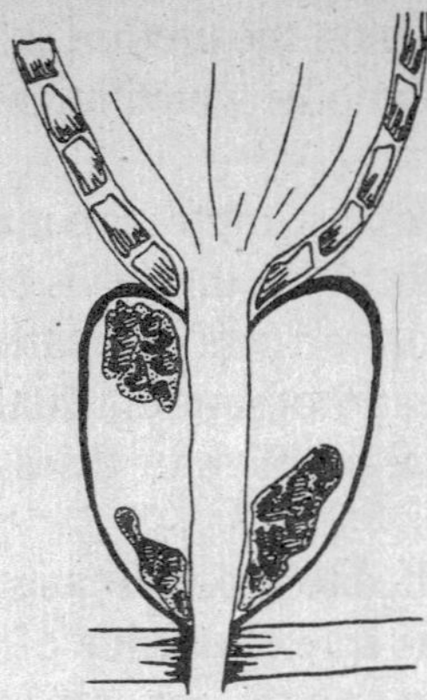

One urologist says he shows the patient the device and the noise it will make. During the actual biopsy the patient jumps when he hears the sound, not because of pain. For most the use of the biopsy gun is quick, simple and painless. A lot easier than going to the hospital for a biopsy the old way. And that means it's less costly as well for the patient.

One patient said it was less painful for him than a shot in the arm, like a flu shot.

The tissue core taken in the biopsy is evaluated to see if it is cancerous.

Another technique known as fine-needle aspiration cytology is often used these days. Here a urologist inserts an extremely fine needle through the rectum and removes cells from the prostate in three, four or five different locations. The technique results in minimum pain for the patient and no anesthesia is required.

If the tissue shows evidence of cancerous growth, the urologist usually will do more testing. This is to find out the placement of the cancer and the extent of it. One of these tests is the PSA test, the prostate specific antigen test. If the prostate is producing a higher level of antigen than usual, it is a good indication that cancer is present.

The other test, the PAP, or the prostate acid phosphatase, may reveal if the cancer has spread to other parts of the body. If the PAP is elevated, the urologist will follow up with chest X-rays and X-rays of the pelvic area as well as bone scans and perhaps a CAT scan if equipment is available.

There is another way that many men learn that they have cancer of the prostate. This happens during a routine TURP operation where BPH has resulted in an operation. The scrapings of tissue from the prostate are examined to see if they are benign or cancerous. If the pathologist reports there are some flakes that show cancer, the doctor then does more tests to determine the placement of the tumor, and the chance that he has already removed all of the cancerous tissue.

When cancer is found in this instance, it is usually an early beginning of the disease, and one that was not found, or was not in the right place to be discovered, with the digital exam.

Again here more tests would be done and the prostate examined again to determine what procedure might be needed. This would be after the regular BPH surgery, since most evaluations of prostate tissue by a pathologist take two to three days in most areas on a routine basis.

Can Cancer of the Prostate Be Cured?

The quicker it can be diagnosed and treated, the better the chances are for cure.

Any cure depends on the treatment, so that's the next

thing your urologist will look at. What will work best for this type and size of cancer on this patient considering his general health, his wishes and his age?

Urologists classify cancers in four stages, A, B, C, and D.

Stage A:

In stage A cancer it is silent, the patient doesn't know he has it. It can't be felt by digital rectal examination or even suspected for any reason. A PSA test here might show up the elevated antigen and lead to a suspicion. This is one reason many people are suggesting that PSA tests be given to every man over forty years of age as a part of his annual physical.

The stage A of cancer is almost always found when a TURP or other operation is carried out for BPH. The removed prostate tissue examined by a pathologist will show evidences of cancer.

Stage B:

Stage B cancer is usually detected as a lump or hard or firm area on the prostate's two outer lobes during a digital rectal examination. This might be after a man has reported BPH symptoms, or during a routine physical.

Stage C:

In stage C the cancer is usually found by digital rectal exam or after a BPH caused exam. Here much and sometimes all of the prostate that can be felt is hard and firm indicating the cancer. At this stage the cancer probably has spread from the prostate itself into the immediate vincinity.

Stage D:

In stage D the cancer has spread from the prostate into any of the adjoining body areas such as the lymph nodes. By this time the cancer may also have spread into the lungs, or bones or any part of the body.

Treatment for the Four Stages of Cancer

Stage A Prostate Cancer

Prostate cancer here is usually a surprise to the doctors and to the patient since there were no symptoms or any way it could be detected. Usually it is found during an operation for Benign Prostatic Hypertrophy, BPH.

The pathologist would make the find and report to the physician indicating the amount of cancerous tissue found and if possible the type and seriousness of the cancer.

Here there are two distinct types of cancer. One is fairly nonaggressive. In eighty-five percent of these cases of stage A cancer, the patient is totally relieved of his small "starting" cancer. He is cured and never bothered by any return of prostatic cancer again.

However in the other fifteen percent of the cases, the cancer is a vigorous type and must be treated with all possible haste. Some patients in this group will have a rapid development of the cancer and succumb to the disease in a short time. Treatment here should be as vigorous as with stage B cancer.

Stage B Prostate Cancer

This stage of cancer development is the type that is found by digital examination. This is the usual way to discover it, since there are no outward physical symptoms, hurts or even twinges. The cancer is still silent.

This is why it's so vital for every man over forty years of age to have a rectal digital examination at least once a year. Three minutes isn't too much to give up for saving your life.

Stage B cancer shows up as a hard nodule or lump or ridge that the urologist will confirm. Most experts in the field say that at this stage the cancer is curable. Catching it at this early stage is the one lifesaving factor.

Once the cancer has been diagnosed, its extent is then determined by the various examinations such as a PSA test, bone X-rays, bone scans and a PAP test.

Often at this point the nearby lymph nodes will be removed to be sure that the cancer has not spread into them. If the cancer is confined to the prostate, the most used treatment is the complete removal of the prostate gland.

Stage C Prostate Cancer

In stage C almost the entire prostate has been invaded by and taken over by the cancerous cells. Again cancer in this stage does not produce any notice to the victim that anything is wrong. Cancer is still silent here, so again, every man must appreciate the value and the lifesaving importance of a digital examination at least once a year.

The digital examination is the only way that this cancer can be detected, with the exception of a PSA test. Many urologists do not give PSA tests except when cancer is already expected. It seems reasonable that the PSA test should be given all men over the age of forty as a secondary cancer screening test.

The stage C cancer is still treatable because it has not spread to other parts of the body. Early detection again is the key here to living.

The lymph nodes should be examined by a CAT scan to be sure the cancer hasn't spread. With a negative report, the usual course is radiation or hormonal treatment. When this is done, the patient's cure is possible, but there is a chance that some of the cancer cells have escaped into the lymph nodes or other areas of the body. A cure for stage C prostate cancer is not as good as with stages A and B.

Stage D Prostate Cancer

When the cancer has spread widely beyond the confines of the prostate capsule, it is called a stage D cancer. Again, this cancer may not have any symptoms the unsuspecting man can feel soon after it spreads into other areas. If the cancer has spread into the bones there may be severe pain. If so, this will cause the patient to seek help from his physician.

Generally stage D prostate cancer is not curable but it can be supressed. If it has spread only to the lymph nodes around the prostate, there is a chance that with vigorous treatment the cancer can be contained and the patient have a longer survival.

Urologists differ on what treatment to give a patient at this point. Some say if the cancer has spread into bones and lungs and other parts of the body, it is probably incurable, therefore radical surgery is not called for and hormonal treatment should be used.

A few urologists say with minor spreading of the cancer a radical prostatectomy (removal of all of the prostate) and a bilateral orchiectomy (removal of both testicles) is the proper course. The testicles are removed because at least ninety percent of all prostate cancers are encouraged to grow with the presence of the male hormone.

The androgens help the cancers to grow. By removing them from the body the cancer growth may be slowed or stopped. Here there is no agreement among urologists about this type of operation since it is used basically to make the patient feel better.

A new drug out is said to do much the same thing that the removal of the testicles does. It is administered by injection once a month and lowers the levels of the testosterone. When this happens doctors say that the tumor can shrink, relieving some of the pain and other symptoms.

"Zoladex offers patients a safe and effective alternative to the traditional therapies in the treatment of advanced prostate cancer," according to Mark E. Soloway, urologist and chief of urologic oncology at the University of Tennessee.

Nothing was said about the side effects, but with sufficient use to shrink the testicles, there would also probably be sterilization and impotency as well.

Many scientists believe that prostate tumors, like others, may manufacture their own growth hormone. A new drug called Suramin is now being used to try to suppress and eliminate that growth hormone. More testing is being done. A group of thirty men at the National Cancer Institute in Bethesda, Maryland underwent a test with the drug. All had prostate cancer, and many of those in the program reported a dramatic decrease in pain from the cancer.

Cancer of the prostate is on average an older man's disease. Yet most doctors and urologists will not do radical surgery on a man over seventy years of age, unless there are special circumstances. The feeling by most urologists is that cancer in older men grows slowly. A seventy-year-old man probably will live just as long with or without the surgery for cancer. As with any medical procedure there are always exceptions to this general rule.

Some radiation therapy is used after prostate surgery to destroy a few cancer cells that might have been missed. However chemotherapy is usually not of much value to the stage D prostate patient.

Usually when the cancer has spread beyond the prostate and is in an active stage in several other areas, no prostate surgery is done, since it wouldn't cure the problem, and could cause other dangers to the patient.

With the stage D patient, the most the physician can do is lessen his pain and do treatments that will make the patient feel better both physically and psychologically.

Radiation Treatment

We mentioned briefly radiation therapy as a treatment for cancer of the prostate. This is simply the use of radiation aimed at a specific part of the body where the cancer cells are in an effort to kill them.

Radiation therapy has developed greatly since it was first used in the early 1920's. Now radiation therapy is often used in combination with other types of treatments.

The traditional method is the use of an external radiation beam aimed at the prostate from outside the body. Sometimes this beam touches the rectum and bladder causing distressing side effects. Some radiation treatments of this type require the patient to come to the doctor's office every day for seven weeks.

A new development in the last few years in radiation is the use of what is called "seed implantation." Here small pelletized radiation charged "seeds" are implanted directly in the cancerous tissue. This can be done on an outpatient basis and usually requires only one trip.

It takes about an hour and utilizes a local or general anesthesia. The urologist, using ultrasound as a guide, projects the patient's prostate on a video screen, locates the tumor and then implants the radiation seeds precisely throughout the prostate to kill the cancerous tumors. A radiation oncologist is a member of this surgical team.

The tiny radiation seeds are inserted through the skin directly into the prostate. There is no incision.

One of the advantages with implantation is that the use of radiation seeds mean there is little or no damage to healthy tissue. The radiation affects only the cancer in the prostate, eliminating any side effects on the rectum or bladder.

These tiny seeds radiate into the prostate for seventeen to thirty-five days. After that time they become used up and "inert." During these days of radiation, the cancer tumor is destroyed, it shrinks and the dead tissue is gradually absorbed and passed off by the body.

Radiation seeds are most effective against the early stages of prostate cancer, A and B. Since cancer in this gland has no early warning signs, men need to be sure they are examined digitally once a year, or with blood tests. If there is any question by the physician, the patient should consult a urologist for further tests such as ultrasound. Early detection is the key to surviving prostate cancer.

One side effect of radiation either internal or externally applied, is fatigue. Even with this problem, many men are still able to go about their jobs and their non-physical work while being given radiation treatments. From time to time a patient given external radiation will have a skin reaction where the radiation passed through.

These reactions can be reduced if the patient avoids using strong soaps, heat lamps, and hot water bottles as well as cologne. If the skin becomes flaky, itchy or red, cornstarch can be used as a powder that will sooth the patient.

Cryosurgery

Since the first part of 1992, a new form of treatment for prostate cancer has been the use of cryosurgery. Two or three specialists refined the method of using intensely cold liquid nitrogen to free up and kill the sections of the prostate where cancer had been detected.

In an issue of the *Cancer Communications* newsletter published by PAACT, the nationwide cancer patients' advocate group, the procedure functions like this: five cryoprobes are inserted into the prostate to freeze and destroy the epithelial cells of the prostate.

With the use of transrectal ultrasound, the doctor can view the placement of the five thin probes and judge the use of the freezing probes. The probes are inserted through the skin midway between the scrotum and the anus under a general anesthesia. No radical incision is made, which means a quicker recovery.

Many patients leave the hospital after 48 hours with only minor discomfort and require no long healing process.

The procedure is completed in about three hours with little discomfort.

Ideal patients for this type of cancer surgery are those with A and B prostate cancer. The hope here is that the cancer can be killed before it can spread to other parts of the body.

During the freezing of the prostate, a heated probe is inserted into the urethra through the prostate to protect it from the freezing.

Normal urination resumes soon after the freezing. Cryosurgery has a better track record concerning sexual potency than prostatectomy. The nerves that control erection at the edges of the prostate are usually not damaged by the freezing. Recent studies show that 60 percent of patients who were potent before the operation return to full potency.

Cryogenic treatment of cancer is in the early stages, but the new cancer treatment gives the patient and doctor another treatment approach to consider.

Dr. Israel Barken of San Diego is also working with the new system and he says it is extremely interesting. He says that the cryogenic treatment of prostate cancer may be the preferred method for dealing with the disease in the future.

Laser Surgery

A continuing study on laser surgery on the prostate

began in 1989 at the University of California at San Diego by Dr. Israel Barken as an alternative to radical prostatectomy. At the time, it was considered an option for patients who were not candidates for open surgery.

Writing in the *Cancer Communication* newsletter, Dr. Barken said that now the techniques of laser surgery have been expanded and defined. Dr. Barken said that there has been limited work done with the laser for prostate cancer because it was felt that this cancer can be in several places in the prostate and the best way to eradicate the disease is to take out the whole prostate.

It was thought impossible to destroy the prostate completely with the laser. In Oslo, Norway, Dr. Hans Beisland developed a technique for treating cancer of the prostate by removing most of the prostate by electrical wire resection, or TURP. Six weeks afterward he systematically used the laser to destroy the remaining tissue.

Since then, Dr. Barken and surgeons in the Institute of Urology of London have started treating patients with prostate cancer using the same two-step approach. The number of patients has been limited due to the technical problems of applying the laser in an accurate manner.

The development of the new 90-degree firing laser now makes it possible to skip the TURP electrical wire resection and "blow out" a cavity inside the prostate with the laser. Then, after six weeks, the laser is again applied to the remaining shell of the prostate from the inside to kill and remove any leftover cancer cells.

This procedure is done on an outpatient basis, with a catheter left in for only one day. The ability to use ultrasound as a guidance to the laser cutting is another step forward in the laser surgery of the prostate.

In the future, lasers may be used more often on prostate cancer. There are new types of laser fibers that can be inserted inside the prostate itself to treat a cylinder of tissue. The combination of rectal ultrasound and the multiple laser interstitial application makes the procedure more exact.

Laser surgery generally has several advantages for the patient:

- It involves little or no pain.
- It can be done without anesthesia, or with only local anesthesia.
- It results in no bleeding.
- It takes little time to complete.
- It can be repeated several times without ill effects, and it can also be done in stages.
- It may be done in a doctor's office or on an outpatient basis at a hospital.

Hormone Treatments

The male hormone, produced mainly in the testes, helps the growth of prostate cancer. One of the radical surgeries removes both testicles to eliminate the male hormone in a man's system.

If the patient can't stand such an operation physically or psychologically, the same result can be obtained by the use of female hormones . . . estrogen. This often is a small pill called DES and the dosage is three milligrams a day.

As with the testicle removal, DES will reduce most

men's libido and prevent them from having an erection. A man's breasts may also enlarge. There may also be a slower growth of beard and some small changes in a man's bodily shape.

To many men, these small changes may be worthwhile if the treatment will help to control or even stop the growth of the cancer, and mean they have another one or two or ten years of life.

Chemotherapy

Chemotherapy is thought of by the general public as a cancer only type of treatment. Actually, any chemical used as a treatment, even an aspirin, is chemotherapy.

With cancer, chemotherapy is a method of killing cancer cells. Unfortunately while killing the bad cells, it also kills and harms a lot of good cells.

While chemotherapy is a major treatment for some kinds of cancer, it is not as effective in prostate cancer. However there are new drugs and new combinations of drugs being developed all the time, and in the future some chemotherapy might work miracles.

For now, chemothrapy for prostate cancer is rarely used. The benefits would not offset the side effects which include hair loss, chronic fatigue, nausea and a general feeling of sickness and depression.

Immunotherapy

With this treatment, the physician attempts to build

up a patient's natural defenses against all diseases, including cancer. The immune system is a complicated mechanism and science is learning more about it all the time.

Immunotherapy is now being combined with some kinds of chemotherapy to treat the more advanced stages of some cancers. One of the elements now being used is Interferon, which comes to light now and again as a breakthrough in treatments. Then it settles back into a low profile, until it is thrust up again. It may yet be developed into a potent cancer fighter.

Quackery Incorporated

Every few years desperate patients try everything suggested by urologists and oncologists and nothing stops their cancer. Suddenly they hear about a new miracle cure for cancer and take off for Mexico or Italy or Spain to get this new wonder drug.

One such hot item in recent memory was Laetrile made from the pits of apricots. For two or three years there were glowing testimonials how it had cured or put into remission cancers of all types.

The product was never approved for sale in the United States and smuggling it across the Mexican border became big business. Clinics sprang up quickly in border towns on the Mexican side where men of questionable qualifications and ethics prescribed and distributed Laetrile to thousands who came to the clinics. They all hoped that Laetrile would cure them. It didn't.

The National Cancer Institute said quickly that Laetrile was useless, that it was a toxic cyanide laden product that could cure nothing and could cause harm.

New "miracle cures" will pop up every few years as long as there are cancer patients who can't be cured.

Most of these quackery medications do no harm—of themselves. The big problem and tragedy, is that they take the cancer patient away from legitimate medical care and put him in the hands of the unscrupulous or the self-healer, and the victim does not get the care that may have some chance to stop or slow or even cure the cancer.

Prostate Cancer, The Outlook

Somewhere near 100,000 men in this country will develop prostate cancer this year. Of that number about 28,000 will die from the disease. Prostate cancer is the third leading cause of men's cancer death in the United States.

What You Should Do

- If you're over 50 years of age, insist on a digital rectal examination of your prostate yearly.
- Also get a PSA test at the same time even if you have to pay the $50 extra for it to be done. It could reveal cancer in your prostate that the finger didn't find.
- Recognize the early signs of an enlarged prostate. If these symptoms come on suddenly, say over a three to six month period, see your physician at once. It might be cancer of a virulent and aggressive kind, and not just BPH.

- Remember that the best way to whip cancer of the prostate is to catch it early. Don't forget about it. Every time your wife has a mammogram, remember that you should have your prostate examined.

8

Can I Still Have Sex After Prostate Trouble?

This probably will be the most read chapter in the book, and rightly so. The prostate is tightly bound up with a male's manhood, and how he thinks of himself as a man. That's why even the mention, let alone the discussion, of the prostate and its troubles, make most men uneasy, nervous and embarrassed.

We'll look at all problems with the prostate and how they may or may not affect a man's libido, his attitude, his sexual performance and his sexual desires.

Prostatitis and Sex

The first problem many men have with their prostate is prostatitis. Symptoms of this involve lower back pain, pelvic discomfort, a burning in the penis when urinating, urinary frequency and sometimes a slight pain after ejaculation.

This form of noninfectious prostatitis may be caused by some infectious agent we know nothing about, or by some noninfectious form of inflammation. On the other hand, it also can be caused by a man's sexual habits—too much sex or too little.

During arousal, a man produces four times the prostatic fluid he usually does. If this fluid is not discharged by ejaculation, it remains in the prostate. If this happens often, the prostate can become seriously congested.

To prevent this problem, a normal, healthy sex life is the best course of action. If this is not possible, a massage of the prostate by a urologist will relieve the congested prostate and eliminate the pain. If that's not desired, masturbation is a quick solution suggested by many urologists.

Too much sex, too quickly, say eight or ten ejaculations in a two day period, can overwork the prostate and again cause problems. On the other hand, abstinence may cause a build up of prostatic fluids and lead to congestion so a massage is needed.

Coitus interruptus, simply the removal of the penis before ejaculation, is a method of birth control once practiced by millions. If done often enough, and if it stops the man's climax, this too, can lead to an oversupply of fluid in the prostate and bring about congestion and its symptoms.

If coitus interruptus is used frequently by a couple, the man or woman should continue to excite the penis to a normal ejaculation to prevent buildup problems in the prostate.

So for prostatitis, which can strike men of any age, sexual intercourse may be both the cause and the solution.

Infectious Prostatitis

This inflammation of the prostate is caused by some type of infection and can cause fever, chills, nausea and vomiting as well as an urgency to urinate, burning, pain and blood and pus in the urine. It's more serious than the noninfectious type.

There may be serious congestion of the prostate and urologists sometimes use a prostate massage to relieve it. Most urologists feel that sexual activity of any type that leads to ejaculation is the ideal way to empty the prostate and relieve the congestion.

Benign Prostatic Hyperplasia

With the enlargement of the prostate there will be some sexual changes, particularly if there is surgery involved.

As you may remember, a man will have a normally enlarging prostate for ten to fifteen years, maybe more, before he notices it. The enlargement itself does little to sexual performance with the exception of a seriously pinched urethra that could reduce the amount and force of an ejaculation.

When it comes to needed surgery for BPH, the question of sex becomes more important.

First, there should be no sexual intercourse for six weeks after a normal TURP surgery. This is to allow time for the "canal" dug through the enlarged prostate tissue to heal.

On a standard TURP operation to remove enlarged prostate tissue, about six percent of all men operated on will become impotent. That means they will not be able to have a normal erection.

There are bundles of nerves on each side of the prostate, and some of these control the impulses and nerve responses that combine to produce an erection. If these nerve bundles are damaged in any way, impotence can follow.

Remember, this six percent figure may not be totally accurate. The figure is based on subjective information supplied by the patient. It wouldn't be unusual for a man 68 or 70 or older to claim that he could have an erection before the operation, when in reality he had lost that ability due to natural aging or some other problem.

It is a factor to consider.

The other change in a man who has had a TURP operation is that the bladder neck may have been damaged or removed during the TURP. The bladder neck is like a "valve" that automatically closes when a man is ejaculating. It prevents the fluids from going upward into the bladder. The urethra muscles then force the fluid out the end of the penis.

After a TURP operation, the bladder neck may no longer be there or it may be enlarged to such an extent that the fluids of the ejaculation take the path of least resistance, and flow upward a half inch or so and empty into the bladder.

When this happens the man has *exactly the same physical sensations* that he had when the ejaculate emptied out the end of his penis. The feeling, the motion, the thrill is the same, only the path the fluid takes is different. This retrograde ejaculation is almost a one hundred percent probability in a TURP or open surgery for BPH. It's simply a fact of life. However, with men who usually are in the operative stage, their age is often in the early to late sixties or later, and the lack of a penile ejaculation does not present much of a problem. This is especially true if the situation is carefully explained to the patient and his wife *before the operation*.

Cancer of the Prostate

Stage A and B cancer of the prostate will usually involve a radical prostatectomy, the complete removal of the prostate. This almost always harms the nerve bundles on both sides of the prostate and results in a man being impotent. However new techniques have now been developed to preserve these nerves. Some urologists say that in so doing, they may leave some cancer cells behind after the operation.

At this point the cancer is the main concern, the life of the patient, and not his sexual function. The surgeon will try his best to get all of the cancerous growth. The nerve bundles are not a high priority.

For the man who might be in his fifties, and is cured of a stage A cancer of the prostate, there are drugs and devices that can help him achieve an erection for satisfying intercourse.

The cancer patient who is treated with radiation, internal or external, can usually continue his sex life without any problems. His sexual ability would be the same before or after the radiation with the exception of the normal radiation caused fatigue problems. When used in certain areas, radiation can also cause impotence.

For the cancer patient with stage D cancer of the prostate, which is usually not operable, the man's sex life would be in direct relation to where the cancer was situated and how it affected his ability to perform. At this point the patient is much more interested in extending his life, and not worried about his sexual function.

Some Drugs Can Defeat Impotence

There are drugs that can be used to help an impotent man. One of them is called papaverine, and many urologists suggest its use. The drug is injected directly into the side of the penis. This drug causes a dilation of arteries in the penis thereby increasing the flow of blood to the penis and also causes less blood to leave the penis.

Blood is what causes an erection, and with the increased flow, many impotent men are able to achieve a firm erection and subsequent intercourse.

The patient is given the first injection in the office to teach him how to do it. A skinny needle is used and there is no pain involved. The medication will cause a temporary burning sensation but it's not severe.

Sometimes a patient has psychological problems involved with his impotence. Papaverine is especially good in these cases. By injecting himself, the patient achieves and maintains an erection for up to an hour. This will naturally reduce the fear of failure which results so often in a poor performance anxiety.

Some urologists gradually reduce the dosage and frequency of the shots. For patients with purely psychological impotency problems this can result in a return to normal sexual function without any shots.

Another drug, Prostaglandins, is also being used for penile injections to help in impotency. It is also a vein-dilating medication and works much the same way that Papaverine does.

What about the over the counter aphrodisiacs that can be found in many health food stores? Most aren't labeled as such, but the advertising or the labels suggesting a vigor for life, and an elixir especially for men, tell what they are selling.

The Food and Drug Administration has simply banned all aphrodisiacs from sale with the explanation that they do not do what they claim. Most still sold don't help, but don't do that much harm either. Here you have to remember the placebo effect. If a sugar pill will help a man to get a workable erection, use it and don't ask questions.

One old folk remedy, however, is being talked about by some serious researchers and physicians. This is yohimbine. It comes in a pill form and some doctors say it can help restore function and desire in some men. It is said to dilate blocked blood vessels and helps in the release of norepinephrine. Doctors say this compound is helpful in causing and maintaining erections. We expect to hear more about this yohimbine in the years ahead.

Prostheses

For more than twenty years now, there have been available to urologists mechanical penile prostheses to implant in patients who are impotent.

Today there are several types available and the man who can't achieve a firm erection and can't achieve penetration, may want to talk to his urologist about such a mechanical device.

Before the talks get very far the urologist may suggest that the man and his wife go see a specialist in sexual counseling. Implanting a penile prostheses is a big decision for a couple to make, and before it happens, both partners must be sure this is the right thing to do.

Sometimes a man will go ahead with such a project because he thinks that his wife wants him to. He may go through the operation and the certain amount of pain and recovery time required, only to find that his wife wasn't all that eager for him to do it.

It is best before any commitments are made for the couple to receive qualified counseling, and then to have a frank discussion with their doctor or urologist about the devices available, which would be best for this particular man, how they work, what can go wrong, how much the operation costs, and the end results of the procedures.

A single man of any age, should consider his situation carefully. He may want to consider the effect such an operation might have on his friends, and anyone with whom he is considering having intimate relations. He must ask himself if this is truly something that he wants to do.

When the answer is a "yes" he needs to sit down with his urologist and look over the types of devices available. There are two general types. Those implants which are rigid or semi-rigid and once in place remain the same unless they are removed.

The second type includes those which can be inflated and deflated on demand, that are inflatable or that are hydraulic in nature.

The more recent developments include the inflatable types. Most of these consist of two hollow cylinders. One is implanted on each side of the penis in the area usually filled with blood during a normal erection. These tubes are filled with fluid through the use of a rubber pump that is placed under the scrotum.

This system uses a small pump, a cylinder, a reservoir and interconnecting tubes and every bit of it is concealed beneath the man's skin and can't be seen from the outside.

The abdominal muscles hide the small reservoir and fluid.

To activate this system the man squeezes the pump that forces fluid into the cylinders in the penis, much the way blood does during a natural erection. Some of these models do not require any fluid so have no reservoirs.

To return the penis to a flaccid position, the deflation valve is pushed and the fluid returns to the reservoir and the penis relaxes.

This type of hidden device is more natural, and out of sight, and it permits the penis to return to a normal state when not inflated. The inflated or hydraulic prosthesis is more complicated than some of the others and the most expensive to buy and to have surgically implanted.

The first available device was the Small-Carrion Penile Prosthesis developed by Dr. Michael Small and Dr. Herman Carrion of the University of Miami School of Medicine back in 1970. It is simply a pair of tubes filled with spongy material. They are implanted surgically into the penis and gives a man a semirigid penis that can achieve vaginal penetration.

One of the problems here is that it is the same all the time. A semirigid penis can be embarrassing at times, as well as being uncomfortable.

A later development is made with flexible silicone rods that are hinged for better concealment. Such an implantation allows the penis to hang down normally. It offers a man intercourse but there may be some difficulty in vaginal penetration. The permanent erection here is not quite so hard to live with and the man can wear tight clothing without any undue embarrassment.

The rigid and semirigid implants are the most simple to place, and since they have no working parts, can't break down or malfunction. They are also the least costly but, at the same time, are the most difficult to live with since they leave the penis in a semirigid state 24-hours a day.

None of these prostheses have any bearing on or create any effect on normal urination for the man using them.

A New Idea

A new device is now on the market to help men achieve a workable erection. It's called an Erect Aid Suction Device For Potency. The principal the device uses is that nature hates a vacuum. It's always trying to fill up a partial vacuum.

The device uses a long hollow tube that will fit over a penis. It is fixed to the body with a salve to create an air tight seal and then it is simply held in place with hand pressure.

Then a small pump is used to exhaust the air in the tube. This reduces the pressure inside the tube and blood from the body rushes into the penis to try to fill that vacuum. In doing, it fills the two cavities in the penis and creates an erection. Next the tube is removed and a rubber device is quickly fitted around the base of the penis to retain the blood in place.

The erection will hold for thirty minutes, at which time the band must be removed to let the blood leave. Cost, about $300. This item is available at medical supply houses with a doctor's prescription. There is no injection, no implantation, no mechanical device, no continuing prosthesis that gets in the way, no pain, and it's simple and easy to use. Urologists who suggest this system show their patient a video in the office, then let him take the video home to show to his wife. Some offer a demonstration of the device in the office.

Men who use it say it works wonderfully without any high operating cost, embarrasing hardware or surgical procedures.

9

Nutrition and Your Prostate

Most urologists practicing today would agree that nutrition alone can't cure any prostate problem. However, more and more of them are saying that there may be some connection between diet and nutrition and supplemental vitamin and minerals and the causes and treatment of some kinds of prostate troubles.

A well balanced diet will help to sustain a healthy and well functioning prostate.

Much of this diet concern in regards to the prostate, centers around the mineral, zinc.

There has been a lively discourse and advertising and sales promotion over the past few years promoting zinc as a vital element in the prostate and touting zinc additives as a benefit in preventing prostate problems and treating those present.

Zinc is a mineral trace element that is vital to all human beings. However, the amount of zinc needed is surprisingly low.

Research scientists report that an intake of less than 10 milligrams of zinc per day through diet, probably will cause some type of serious disturbances in a man's organs and glands.

Urologists know that zinc is found in high concentrations in the prostate gland and in the seminal fluid. In fact, the prostate contains more zinc than any other organ of the body. Nobody knows why the zinc is there, or exactly what its function is, or how it's utilized by the body.

Neither can scientists show that the addition of zinc in a supplement by mouth will prevent any prostate disease, or help to treat any existing prostate condition.

Many studies have been made dealing with zinc and the human body and with zinc and the prostate. We have been able to find no double blind scientific tests made with patients taking zinc by mouth. Some tests have been done informally and patients reported symptoms of BPH to be improved. However these same patients were getting other treatments for their BPH so no "single differential" was established.

At the same time there could have been some strong placebo effect here, where the patients got better, or perhaps just altered their attitude toward the symptoms, simply because they thought they were getting medicine that would make them better.

Dr. William Fair, a urologist at the Sloan-Kettering Memorial Medical Center in New York City, has made a long study of zinc and the prostate. He has stated that zinc may be important in the prevention of prostatic diseases. He follows this with the countering opinion that the prostate can't pick up and utilize zinc when it is taken by mouth.

He points out that even when the zinc gets into the bloodstream, the prostate can't utilize zinc from the blood. Dr. Fair says that tests have proved that zinc levels are definitely down in men with prostate cancer. It is not known if this is a result of the cancer attacking the prostate, or if the cancer gets a foothold *because the zinc level is low.*

Other experts say the use of zinc as a possible method for preventing prostate problems seems to be growing in this country. It is now a given that zinc is necessary for a proper and healthy prostate, but for many the question remains, how does the prostate absorb or utilize the zinc that it needs?

Some urologists are coming to believe that the researchers may not be entirely accurate in saying that zinc can't be utilized by the prostate when the trace mineral is in the bloodstream. Long term use of zinc sulphate by mouth is now prescribed by some urologists who believe that the zinc can be absorbed from the blood and that it can have beneficial results in preventing and in treating, BPH and prostatitis.

Vitamins are often given with the zinc supplements. These include B-12 and Vitamin E. Some experts say that the zinc-vitamin combination can't shrink the enlarged fibrous and muscle tissue in the prostate, but that they can shrink the enlarged glandular type tissue. This shrinkage has resulted in easier urination, no dribbling and less nocturia for the BPH patient.

All of the urologists who work with and experiment with zinc and vitamin combinations, say that no man should try to undertake any such dietary supplemental program on his own. When these experimental tests are made with zinc the patients are closely monitored with all kinds of controls. If too much of something has been taken, the urologist is there to remedy the situation before any harm is done.

They point out that the proper dosage of zinc is highly critical, and what might be right for one man, might be far too much for another.

If the zinc and vitamin treatment interests you, your first step should be to call your doctor or urologist and talk it over with him. He will put your best physical being and your best interest at the center of his decisions. Talk to him.

What About Foods?

The people who sell additives and special compounds that are said to "be good for a normal operating prostate" extol the special qualities of pumpkin seeds, saw palmetto, golden rod and flaxseed oil. Do they help the prostate? No one has made any reliable tests here that we could find and the old axiom of let the buyer beware is well put to use for these products. Could there be a placebo effect? We hope so. If it works, it works.

A lot of noise is made by some people who are zinc enthusiasts for the prostate and who promote eating foods rich in zinc. These are not hard to find. But the same basic applies. If zinc can't be utilized by the prostate when it is taken in capsule form, can it be utilized from food? No one knows for sure.

Foods high in zinc include nuts, sunflower seeds, wheat germ and bran, milk, eggs, onions, brewer's yeast, almost all of the seafoods, beef liver, meat, lentils, molasses, peas, beans and poultry.

Several of these foods also are high in cholesterol, such as beef liver, seafood and eggs. Cholesterol is often a problem for men in this 40 to 90 age range, so it can be a bit of a dilemma whether to eat them or not.

Nutritionists are quick to point out that just because a food might be high in zinc in its natural state, that's no sign that the food will still retain the zinc when the food is eaten. Over cooking and processing will quickly eliminate most of the zinc from foods.

One urologist says that if you want to be sure to get your minimum daily requirement of zinc at fifteen milligrams, you'll probably have to take zinc supplement pills.

For those who like to get their vitamins that are thought to be beneficial for prostate from foods, there is a shopping list you can rely on.

Orange Juice . . . high in vitamin C. All citrus fruits also are good here as well as tomatoes. Add to the vitamin C producers such items as broccoli, brussels sprouts, cabbage, strawberries and green peppers.

Milk is a fine source for Vitamin D, but also include tuna, sardines, egg yolks, margarine, fish liver oil and salmon.

If it's vitamin E you need, try peanuts, green leafy vegetables such as cabbage, spinach and asparagus, wheat germ, whole grain bread, vegetable oils and rice.

Avoiding certain foods is important for anyone with a

prostatic condition. This bears repeating. Spicy foods, alcohol, coffee and caffeine drinks of all sorts irritate the prostate. If you're really having prostate trouble, your doctor will probably advise you to abstain from all of the above food and drink items.

The proof is not yet available to confirm or deny the value of the use of a special diet or vitamins or zinc supplements with the hope of lessening your prostatic ailments, or of preventing any such problems. Zinc may turn out to be the cure for BPH and a treatment that will do wonders but not yet.

The same is true for vitamins and food supplements: We're not sure what is of value and what can help the prostate.

General health is another matter, so the balancing act here is for the prostate sufferer to maintain a wholesome and balanced diet getting plenty of the basic foods and eating and drinking in moderation.

If you have the idea of self-prescribing a zinc and vitamin and food regimen for yourself, do your body a favor. Go talk to your doctor or urologist about it first, and see what he suggests. After all, he's the doctor.

10

You've Got a Couple of Symptoms . . . What's Next?

All right, you've read this far so you must have some personal interest in this prostate situation. What does the reasonably intelligent man do when he realizes that, by Jupiter, *he does have a couple of those BPH symptoms?*

BPH and a Doctor's Visit

What comes next? If you're married, the first thing you do is talk it over with your wife. She probably knows, but tell her what you've been feeling. Let's say that you're getting up twice at night to go to the bathroom, and a couple of times you almost stopped at a stranger's house because you had to urinate so bad on a car trip and the filling stations were closed.

Besides that, sometimes it takes you ten seconds or so

to get your stream started once you relax and get ready to urinate.

How old are you now? Fifty-eight. Fair enough. You know that your prostate has been growing since you were about fifty. How big is the thing now? Is it causing these wake up calls? Time to find out. If you belong to an HMO or have a private physician, your best bet is to make an appointment and go see him. What he'll probably do is check your medical history to see if you've made this type of complaint before. You probably haven't.

Your doctor now will ask you a lot of questions, some that may seen strange or unrelated, but answer them as truthfully and completely as you can. Many doctors will check your age and your symptoms and will be thinking BPH.

He will work through the entire list of BPH symptoms. How many times do you get up at night to urinate? Do you have trouble sometimes starting your flow? Trouble all the time? Does the stream sometimes stop before you finish voiding and then start again a few seconds later?

He'll want to know if you feel like you've emptied your bladder when you urinate. Can you tell if your stream is weaker now than it was five years ago? This is hard to answer because any diminishing of a urine stream is gradual.

He'll ask you if you have any pain or discomfort when you urinate. When you have the urge to go to the bathroom, must you go at once, or can you hold it to a convenient time? Have you ever dribbled or lost urine involuntarily before or after urinating? Have you ever noticed any blood in your urine?

When you finish answering these questions, your doctor will have a much better idea about your chances of having BPH.

Your doctor will probably ask you about any previous surgery in your pelvic area, or in your urethra, any history of gonorrhea, diabetes or any spinal cord injury. The majority of these problems don't apply to most patients, so usually the diagnosis is looking more and more like BPH.

Many general practitioners at this point will do a digital rectal examination to see what they can find. This is no big deal.

If you're over 40 or 50, you've probably had such a probe during a physical exam. If not, be assured it's simple, quick and not painful. Your doctor will put on a plastic glove and lubricate one finger. He'll have you bend over an examining table and gently insert his finger into your rectum. The prostate gland is right beside a portion of the colon and can be felt by the probing finger.

The doctor will be able to touch only the two lateral lobes of the prostate, but this is usually enough to tell him that your prostate is enlarged and it probably is the cause of your BPH symptoms. The great majority of BPH is caused by these two lobes enlarging.

At this point he'll probably tell you that he felt no lumps, no ridges or hard places in the prostate. This means you probably don't have any prostatic cancer forming in those areas. However, as we have seen earlier, some ten to thirty percent of prostate cancer is without any outward signs at the early stages. Which means that his trained finger can't find it even if it's there. We'll talk more about this.

What your doctor can't tell you positively is that you *don't have BPH.* Even if the lateral lobes don't feel enlarged, the middle lobe he can't feel could be the culprit. Also the lobes could be growing against the urethra at the middle of the prostate and not enlarging outward, thereby causing the BPH symptoms but not feeling enlarged to the examining finger.

Probably your family doctor will now decide that you may have BPH and he wants to refer you to a specialist in this field, a urologist. If you're in an HMO you'll be sent to the urology department where a doctor will talk to you. If your doctor has a private practice, he'll refer you to a urologist in private practice who he's worked with before.

A urologist is a medical doctor who specializes in the urinary tract in men and women and in the reproductive system of men.

If this is your first visit to the urologist there will be an interview where he'll ask you many of the same questions that your family doctor did. Be patient, he's trying to get a good "reading" on you and your condition. After he's satisfied himself that he has all the information from you he can get, he'll probably do a digital exam. His findings will probably be the same as the doctor's but he's the specialist and may find something more.

Next your doctor will probably do a urine analysis to look for white blood cells which could mean infection in the urinary tract.

Blood will be drawn for a blood test before the rectal exam, since this exam can upset certain levels from the prostate. One of the tests will be to check your kidney function. Many urologists will do a PSA test to check on the antigen level in the prostate. If this level is higher than normal, it can be a strong indication that there can be a cancer forming in your prostate. In some cases this test gives false readings, but it is a good one to use at this point for diagnosis.

At this point your urologist will know a lot more about your condition. If your prostate is enlarged, but the symptoms are not severe enough to cause you great distress, your urologist will probably say it's a condition now for you to manage.

Most BPH patients learn to "live with" their symptoms while they are not too severe. Some doctors say getting up once or twice a night and some other minor symptoms of BPH can be lived with, with little pain or irritation.

One urologist said when you are getting up three times a night and have to urinate every two hours during the day, and dribble and it takes you twenty seconds to get your flow started—then you're probably ready for surgery.

Most urologists have two general approaches to BPH. As long as the patient has no major problems living with the symptoms, the doctor is content to examine him regularly and watch the slow progress of the BPH. This might be several years. When the patient has had enough and the symptoms are disruptive enough, then he'll come looking for relief.

On the other hand, if there are indications that the bladder can't be emptied, this can create back pressure on the kidneys and the start of deterioration of the kidney function. In these cases, surgery is needed and rather quickly.

At this point, we'll get back to our 58-year-old man, our typical patient. He had the three minor symptoms of BPH. His urologist confirmed the enlargement, explained the options of surgery or "maintenance" and our patient said he could live with the condition. He was glad to know what caused it, found out he could manage it better by cutting down on drinking alcohol, cut out all caffeine drinks, and by not taking any liquid after four in the afternoon. When he went out to the theatre or some social engagement, he always made sure to urinate just before he left the house.

Our typical patient goes home a happy man, knowing his condition, knowing what causes it, and figuring that he can "maintain" his situation for at least another eight or nine years before the symptoms get so bad he will need surgery to provide him with his desired quality of life.

BPH Surgery Required

Now, let's look at a new problem. You're the new patient and you are 63. You've been living with your BPH for five years and it's getting slowly worse. Then last week you thought you were going to die. You couldn't empty out your bladder. You knew the signs to watch for and made a quick trip to your urologist who has been monitoring your condition for the past five years.

What comes next?

Your doctor is worried about kidney damage from back pressure on them. He suggests a couple of tests. First he'll probably do some tests to see if your bladder is emptying enough to avoid back pressure on your kidneys. Some urologists will use an ultrasound study of the kidneys along with a kidney and bladder scan. Some do special X-rays of kidneys and bladder.

Your tests come up with enough evidence to show that there is definitely too much back pressure and there may be the start of kidney damage so surgery is required. A simple operation to clear out the clogged urethra will probably solve the problem.

If you've been a long time patient, the doctor may have enough information to help you pick the right surgery.

Most BPH surgeries done these days, about 95%, are TURP, the through-the-urethra closed surgery.

For the patient new to the urologist, there are other tests the doctor may want to perform. One is a peak flow rate, the flow of urine at the highest rate during voiding. If this is less than 10 milliliters per second, you probably need surgery. If it is over 20 milliliters per second, the urethra is not the problem.

The other test some urologists make is the cystoscopic examination. This is intra-urethral. It lets the doctor judge if there is any bladder damage, check for bladder tumors, and helps him decide if a TURP operation is the best way to solve the problem for this patient.

Most men will react quickly to the idea of something being inserted through their penis in that small little tube that carries the urine. It's a natural reaction.

But when it's done correctly, there's little pain and it's more the thought of it being done than the actual exam that is the worst part of this procedure for most men.

When any medical tool or catheter is inserted into the urethra there must be anesthetic used. Usually this is an anesthetic jelly squirted into the opening at the end of the penis and forced along the tube. Some men say this is the most painful part. Then the anesthetic does its job of deadening the nerve endings and the pain is over.

When the anesthesia does its work, the instrument is put into the urethral opening at the end of the penis and gently and slowly pressed inward through the penis, past the prostate and into the opening of the bladder.

The urologist will take from three to five minutes for this whole examination. He'll examine the inside of the bladder to be sure there is no disease there or any other problem, then check the interior of the urethra to determine the extent of the blockage.

When the examination is over, the doctor and patient will talk again. Now the urologist will know for sure if he feels that the patient needs surgery.

If there is some danger of kidney damage, such as from urine retention in the bladder, a catheter will be inserted, the urine drained and the catheter left for a few days or a few weeks to see if the kidneys can regain their normal function. If not, an operation will be needed.

So On To Surgery!

The decision is made, your symptoms are too much for you, they're causing pain and intruding on your normal life. Get it done! Many men say they feel a sense of relief once the surgery has been scheduled. A problem that's been dogging them for as much as ten years, is going to be reduced and modified, maybe even eliminated!

You are admitted to the hospital. Now comes more examinations, one to assess your general health and condition. There will be a chest X-ray and an electrocardiogram and basic lab blood work and urine tests and maybe a few more.

The average stay in the hospital for most TURP patients these days is 48 hours. Not long enough to learn your nurse's name!

You'll talk with your anesthesiologist, and may be given your choice of how you get knocked out. Most urologists these days prefer spinal anesthesia. They say this allows the pelvic muscles and those in the abdomen to be more relaxed. Also there are none of the complications with the "putting the patient to sleep" type of anesthesia.

With the spinal type you will feel no pain or any sensations in your lower body through the one to two hour operation. For this one you and your doctor decided on a TURP. After the operation you'll have a catheter in your bladder and out your penis.

Through this three way catheter your surgical area will be irrigated and the fluid and blood removed through another section of the tube. Now, all that remains is the healing of the canal the doctor carved out through your enlarged prostate.

There is little discomfort or pain just after the surgery. Most urologists send their patients home after two days with the catheter removed.

One question that often gets asked. What happens to the tube that was once there, the urethra? It is gone, cut away when the doctor cut out the enlarged prostatic tissue to create the canal. There's no danger or problem. The urine passes through the canal as it did once through the tube. As soon as the canal tissue heals where it has been cut, it will act just like the urethra used to, only now with a lot more room.

Oh, one more caution. Most urologists want the canal to be entirely healed and all scabbing gone before there is any sexual intercourse. That healing process usually takes about six weeks.

Another reminder. There will be a backflow of your semen into the bladder, instead of out your penis as before. Nothing else will have changed, the thrust, the spasm and feeling will all be the same.

What If You Have Prostatic Inflammation?

When you have some of the intense symptoms of an inflamed prostate from infection or some other reason, the first thing you want is relief. But the first thing you'll get is a sit down talk with your urologist who will ask you a whole sheet full of questions that don't seem important to you.

He'll take a detailed medical history of you, ask about your present symptoms, and any past difficulties or diseases of your genitourinary tract.

The doctor will want to hear your "chief complaint," that's the one that got you off your couch and down to the urologist's office.

He'll also want to know: Do you have pain in the area between your scrotum and anus? Pain in your rectum? Pain deep inside your penis? Any burning or discomfort during urination? Has your urine had a foul odor? Any fever with your symptoms? Any other pains? How long have the pains bothered you? Have you had these pains before? How were they treated? Any sign of blood in your urine? Any kidney stones?

Some types of prostatitis can be the results of the patient's sexual habits and performances. For this reason, your urologist will ask you a lot of searching questions about your sex life in an effort to determine if your condition is due to this activity.

Your doctor will probably give you a physical examination. If you are with a urologist, he'll look at your genitourinary system, since that's where the problem is.

He'll ask you to lie on your back and examine your abdomen looking for any lumps, bumps or a spot of pain or tenderness. He'll check for any enlargement of your bladder. He'll examine your genitals looking for any sign of cancer of the testes. When you stand up, he'll check for any abnormalities in your scrotum.

There will be more tests including a digital rectal exam of your prostate, probably a massage of your prostate and urination so the prostatic fluid in your urine can be caught in a glass and tested.

From these and other tests, the urologist will determine if your problem is from infection or some other reason. Then he'll prescribe medication for the infection, or some new type of sexual behavior if your prostate is congested due to some sexual behavioristic reasons.

Yes, to most of us the word "cancer" is frightening. Probably the only word today that is more dreaded is the killer we call AIDS. AIDS is almost always fatal. Cancer used to be, but today hundreds of thousands of cancers are cured or put in total remission every year.

Cancer of the prostate is one of the worst of the cancers around today—because it is so hard to find, to detect. Many times when the cancer is discovered, it has already spread into other parts of the body and can't be stopped.

However, there are four stages of prostatic cancer, and two of them may be totally curable. It all depends how quickly they are found and stopped.

What is ahead for the patient who is diagnosed with cancer of the prostate?

If a patient goes to his doctor with severe pains in his legs and hips and pelvis that are a result of cancer, it's the worst of the worst. However, if the cancer is discovered as the result of a annual physical checkup—and it's a stage A or B cancer, the chances are that it can be totally removed, and the patient will have many, many more years of active, happy life.

Let's take a patient whose doctor finds from a digital exam what he thinks are hard lumps on the lateral lobes of the prostate.

Next, he'll tell the patient that there may be a problem and he'll suggest that the patient go see a urologist. It is the urologist who will make the additional tests needed to confirm or deny the presence of cancer.

He'll do a biopsy to gain a sample of the lump for a pathologist to check to see if it is cancerous or benign. He may also give a PSA test to check to see if there is an elevated antigen level over ten, which puts the patient at a high risk of cancer.

The urologist may use a rectal ultrasound probe to get a sonogram of the patient's prostate. The probe is about twice the diameter of a lead pencil and it's done with the patient lying down and is not painful.

This patient we're using as an example does have cancer. Now the urologist will want to find out if the cancer has spread into other areas of the body. He'll probably do this with bone scans and CAT scans of the lymph nodes.

All of the tests the urologist takes and studies show that this patient has a small tumor on the prostate—but he can discover no other place where the cancer has spread.

Now the patient and urologist will have another talk, and he'll show how he can operate and remove all of the diseased tissue and probably cure the cancer problem.

The two talk over the options. He'll probably tell the patient that a radical prostatectomy is the best. This will remove the entire prostate and the capsule and is a serious "open" operation. However it should remove every bit of the cancer and result in a complete cure.

First will come the removal and examination of the lymph nodes of the pelvis to be sure the cancer has not spread. If it has spread, the prostatectomy will usually not be done. This is a serious operation and will take between three and five hours.

Yes, with this operation there is a hospital stay, some pain and discomfort followed by a period of recuperation. However, this cancer patient is indeed one of the lucky ones—he was completely cured and lived another 27 years, to age 89.

11

Case Histories of Prostate Patients

Over the years, urologists treat hundreds of cases of all types of prostate problems and they say that most of the cases fall into general categories. But every now and then a case will come along that is different.

Let's look at some case histories that more or less fit into the general types, but at the same time are somewhat unusual.

Joseph W., 61, a retired colonel from the U.S. Marine Corps. After his discharge, he and his wife ran a used bookstore for several years and he played a lot of golf. Then one day he realized he was getting up three times a night to go to the bathroom. His wife chided him about his drinking so he quit drinking his usual three beers every night as he watched television.

After that, Joseph still had to get up twice a night. A

year later he was getting up four times a night. He went to his doctor who sent him to a urologist who tested him and together they decided he had an enlarged prostate, and there was no sign of any cancer. A TURP operation would be best.

After the operation, Joseph was home in two days. Two months later he said "everything" was back to normal. He was sleeping through the night now and his sex life was back on track. He said the reverse ejaculation felt exactly the same as it always did and it didn't bother him in the least. He suffered no bad side effects, no incontinence and no impotence. Joseph W. and his wife were one happy couple.

Grant C., 55, a newspaper reporter one day realized he was getting up twice a night to urinate and sometimes his urine stream was slow. He told his doctor about it. He learned for the first time about an enlarging prostate and what it could do. The doctor said there was no sign of cancer and that he should simply moderate his way of life and live with the minor problems.

Grant learned as much about enlarged prostate as he could, talked with a urologist and decided to give up drinking coffee, tea and cola drinks with caffeine in them. He didn't drink beer or alcohol so that was no problem.

Every year on his annual checkup, Grant had the doctor examine him and the doctor said there seemed to be little additional enlargement of the prostate. Grant said his other symptoms such as hesitancy and frequency of urination were about the same. The doctor told him to continue on a "maintenance" program.

After seven years of managing his BPH problem, Grant said that he felt just about the same way he did when it was first diagnosed. He continues to stay away from caffeine, drinks one caffeine-free cola a day, and takes no fluids after six in the evening.

Now after seven years, Grant is still getting up only once a night, and is careful about making sure that he always urinates before leaving the house, especially when going to a movie where a fast paced action film or horror story builds up tension and the need to urinate. He's interested in the new drugs out that may shrink the prostate, and watching the development of the balloon treatment. He's not looking forward to the time when he has to decide what to do when his prostate grows to the point where it can't be managed within reason.

Charles M., 23, a young man who was drafted into the army during the Korean war and took basic training in California far from his native West Virginia. He bragged that he was the biggest stud in his town. He'd had sex with half the women in the county and they lined up for him. The troops didn't know whether to believe him or not.

He boasted that he had celebrated his drafting by having sex at least twice a night for his last 30 days before he was inducted. Three weeks later in the barracks, he was groaning and moaning and complaining. The next morning he went on sick call and the doctor examined him.

His prostate had grown used to the high production rate of fluid to help the sperm on their way during his 30-

day sex spree. Now even after his sudden celibacy his prostate kept right on over producing. The result was his prostate became congested and extremely painful.

The urologist on the army base quickly found the problem and massaged Charles' prostate relieving his congestion and stopping the pain. The urologist said if Charles felt the same problem coming on again he should relieve it with intercourse or masturbation.

Back in the barracks that night Charles had a wild time telling everyone in exacting detail about his problem, how the doctor corrected it and his suggestion about how to relieve it in the future.

Two weeks later the first passes were given to the troops to go to a nearby town for the day and Charles found another way to relieve his prostate.

Cecil U., 28, a motorcycle cop who loved his job. He rode his bike whenever he could, taking double shifts when he was needed. He was single and had as many women as he wanted. When he established a long lasting relationship with a young woman lawyer, he settled down. His sex life was high powered and exciting.

Then one day he exhibited all of the classic symptoms of congestive prostatitis. He developed a lower-back pain, pelvic discomfort, urinary urgency and pain after ejaculation.

His prostate was soft, boggy and filled with fluid but was not enlarged and did not have any hard lumps or nodules. His doctor told him his problem.

After a long conference, they narrowed down the cause of his pain to an overly active prostate. The constant vibration of the motorbike and the high speeds he often had to ride at, stimulated his prostate and it began to produce additional fluid as it would with sexual stimulation.

But the bike ride did not result in ejaculation which would be a relief to the prostate with the expulsion of a large quantity of the fluid. The excess fluid was stored in the prostate and soon caused the problem.

Cecil told his sergeant his dilemma and Cecil was transferred to a patrol car for three months. His symptoms quickly faded and he felt fine again. He went back on the motorbikes, considered the elite of the force in his city, and soon the prostatitis returned.

Cecil talked it over with his live-in woman friend and they decided that it would be best for his health if he made a permanent transfer off the bikes. He did. Three months later he became a detective and soon had his eye on a lieutenant's rating.

Don K., 71, was calm when he heard he had prostate cancer. He had been a bachelor most of his life, married only once when he was about sixty but it didn't last. He was a quiet man, retired, lived alone and spent his whole time collecting stamps and post marks and "round" cancelations from the smallest towns he could find.

He was an expert on stamps, evaluated collections, bought and sold collections and helped young people start their own albums.

His urologist told him the cancer had not advanced a great deal and there was a good chance to stop it if they removed his prostate. In the counseling, Don was told that there was a high percentage chance that this operation would make him impotent.

Don accepted the statement without blinking and said he would think about it and let the doctor know. A week later the urologist became concerned since he hadn't heard from Don. When he could be pinned down, Don admitted that the idea of impotency frightened him more than the cancer.

Don said he would take the offered radiation treatments and chemotherapy rather than the operation to remove his prostate. The radiation treatments had been explained to him, and he was told that there was a chance that the radiation and the chemotherapy might not stop all of the cancer cells and the disease could spread.

Don accepted this risk.

Six months later the cancer had spread to twenty three separate places in his body. Three months later he died.

Fred G., 77, retired landscaper and ex-navy man had a buildup of BPH symptoms twelve years ago when he was 65 and had a TURP. He came through the operation fine with no harmful side effects.

Today he's 77 and his prostate has been growing slowly for twelve years, but his doctor says not to worry. He's a world traveler, widowed, spends his time visiting relatives in foreign countries and his children and grandchildren here at home.

"I might need another operation, but not for a while. Now my only symptoms are a small weak stream sometimes. The rest of the time it's full and strong. So I don't worry.

"Right now I figure I won't need another operation until I have to get another new driver's license. That won't be for four more years when I'm 81."

There was no sign of cancer when Fred had his operation twelve years ago. He's still clear of it today and is checked regularly by PSA and ultrasound.

"I'm happy as a clam with relatives," Fred said.

Marshal J., 57, vice president of a large retail operation. Salary about $150,000 a year. Marshal was a slight, smaller man of no more than 145 pounds. He was sharp, intelligent, friendly, and on the fast track to the top of his firm as soon as the president and founder figured out that 75 was too old to be running the big chain store.

When Marshal was 55, he had his required company physical and passed with better than average findings. He didn't smoke or drink, played tennis and golf, and was slim and trim. His cholesterol was even within bounds.

When he was 56 he missed his checkup because he was vacationing in Hawaii and just never got it rescheduled. When he was 57 his doctor found hard lumps on his prostate. A biopsy showed them to be malignant.

Marshal and his wife listened carefully to the urologist's talk, looked at the diagrams and weighed the chances. All of the advantages of a prostatectomy operation were laid out for them. The doctor said at this stage he thought it would be a better idea to do a retropubic prostatectomy with an incision.

The doctor explained that to be sure to get all of the cancer they would have to remove so much of the prostate that the bundles of nerves controlling erection would be gone and Marshal would be impotent.

Marshal shrugged, said it was better than being dead in a year. His wife asked him if he was sure. They left the office talking about it. The next morning Marshal called and told the doctor to schedule the operation he thought was the best that would get all of the cancer.

The open surgery was done and the urologist thought that he removed all of the growth, but only time would tell them for sure. There was no way to be sure that the cancer had not already spread to other parts of Marshal's body.

Five years later, Marshal collected the five dollar bet he had made with the urologist during Marshal's regular checkup. The cancer had not spread and had not reoccurred. Marshal and his wife had made the decision that saved his life. He worked with his doctor and selected a penile prostheses, and is happy.

Bob M., 48, A high pressure businessman who was an expert at solving big business problems. He was at the height of his career, had a beautiful house, a lovely wife and a daughter.

He noted some changes in his urination, a slowing and sometimes hesitancy, but figured he was almost fifty and that was just a part of growing old. That was Bob's mistake.

Six months later after a tough business conference, one of his legs began to hurt. The next morning it had swollen and was extremely painful. He went to see his doctor. That afternoon he was referred to a urologist.

The urologist said Bob had the type of prostate cancer that was extremely aggressive. This type brings on BPH symptoms swiftly, perhaps in 6 months the BPH symptoms will be as severe as they might be with normal prostate growth in ten years.

The swelling and pain came from cancer that had quickly left the prostate and spread into his bones and legs and lymph glands.

Bob fought the cancer with all of his strength, angry because here was a problem that needed solving and somehow he didn't have the right answers to solve it.

He grew worse and worse, and at last he realized that the doctors didn't have the answers either. About a year after he was first diagnosed as having cancer, Bob died.

In the last few months of his life, Bob and his wife established a foundation for cancer research that is a viable and progressive organization today in California. His wife hopes that Bob's foundation can find the answer to prostate cancer and save thousands of other fathers and husbands around the world.

Jake A., 73, an ex U.S. navy chief who had retired and was living the good life. He went to his urologist complaining that he had to get up to urinate twice a night and asking what pill he could take to stop it. The urologist explained to him about BPH and said they should do some tests to see if it was time to consider having a TURP operation. Jake admitted that he never could empty his bladder and it gave him a strange feeling. He said he'd get back to the doctor for more tests in a week.

Ten years later when this same Jack A. was 83 years

old, he went back to the same urologist for the tests. By then he was getting up four times during the night, had serious urine retention in his bladder and his peak flow was about three milliliters, not the twenty that would be more normal, and he had a serious dribbling problem when he couldn't hold his urine. His prostate had enlarged to the point where a transurethral resection could not be done.

The more complicated and longer recuperative operation was done, the suprapubic. Jake was in the hospital for a week and a half and had a long recovery. Jake now tells his friends with BPH not to wait too long the way he did to have something done.

Delbert B., 82, was rushed to his urologist's office in an ambulance complaining of severe lower abdominal pain. He had chills and a temperature and he couldn't urinate. The urologist soon found the problem and put a catheter into his bladder through his urethra and took out a large amount of urine.

The chills and fever subsided but the doctors left the catheter in. Later that day the urologist talked to him and he said that he'd never had any trouble urinating, no hesitation, no getting up nights, none of the typical symptoms of BPH.

The urologist took the man's wife into his office and talked to her. She said Delbert would never admit to any kind of problem. She said he had been getting up almost every hour during the night to go to the bathroom. His stream wasn't a stream at all but a five minute series of drips and squirts. She said often she found his urine soiled underwear and pants where he became incontinent.

Another talk with Delbert got to the truth. After several examinations it was determined that he had an advanced case of BPH with a large prostate. They decided his general health and age made him a poor candidate for surgery, even a TURP.

The result was that Delbert was given an indwelling tube into his bladder through his penis to a bag attached to his leg for urine drainage. Delbert used the indwelling tube for another six years until he died of a heart attack. Another case of a man who waited too long, and put up with pain and discomfort for too many years until the problem couldn't be corrected.

Maurice W., 72, had a TURP operation and the pathologist found a few chips in the prostate scrapings that indicated an early cancer.

Maurice's doctor told him about the cancer scrapings but evidently in language that the patient didn't fully understand. Maurice's urination was almost back to normal and he was pleased. The doctor must have decided that the patient was too old and that the slow growing cancer would not create a problem for him. Maurice was not in the best of health having problems with gout and uremia. Here, the doctor decided for the patient that the cancer could be ignored.

Almost no doctor will do this, but in this case the medical expert felt it was justified.

Maurice's other ailments cleared up and about a year later he went to Dr. Israel Barken for a consultation about how he could improve his sex life. When he came he brought with him his medical file from the other doctor. While leafing through the old file, Maurice saw the pathologist's report and picked out the words "malignant neoplasm."

Maurice showed the report to Dr. Barken and asked him what that meant. Dr. Barken told him it meant cancer and they did some examinations at once.

They found irregular hard lumps on Maurice's prostate. A PSA test that showed the antigen level was up to over a value of twenty. A rectal ultrasound probe showed there to be significant cancer in the prostate.

After a consultation with the patient, Dr. Barken suggested radiation treatment might be best for him and he agreed. After a series of radiation treatments the cancer was killed and Maurice is now in his 74th year and enjoying his daily golf game and swimming in his pool.

Walter G., 49, a plumber by trade, met his urologist at the emergency room of a hospital. He complained that he hadn't urinated for two days and felt like he was going to explode. A catheter quickly drained off 500 cc's of residual urine and at once Walter felt better.

In an hour he was joking about how both he and the urologist were in the plumbing business. Then he sobered and asked just what kind of operation did he need so this wouldn't happen again. He called it a "total replumbing of the house." He was concerned about the cost, didn't know if his insurance would cover it, but was determined to get himself fixed the right way.

In a long talk, the urologist took a medical history on

Walter and asked him about any medications he was on. He insisted that he wasn't taking any kind of prescriptions, he was healthy as a horse.

His wife reminded Walter about his three day cold. Then he remembered a specific cold remedy that he had taken. The urologist smiled. He told Walter he wasn't positive but the cold remedy had probably been what caused his problem. The drugs in the pills could have constricted the urethra somehow, shutting off the urine.

The urologist told Walter never to take that cold remedy again or any that had the same drugs in it. After a week Walter called and said he felt great. After a month he was entirely normal with no urination problems.

A big name brand cold remedy had done it. This urologist made a friend for life.

Clyde D., 66. Every urologist has a patient now and then who simply won't face reality. This one was named Clyde and he came in for a simple BPH problem. He was getting up twice a night and knew about the condition, even the name and what was happening. He was a well informed man.

He said it had been two years since he'd had an examination and decided it was time to check out his prostate. A rectal exam revealed one small lump and Clyde was told about it. The urologist said why didn't they do a biopsy right then while he was there with a skinny needle. It would hardly hurt at all and it would save the man a trip.

Clyde refused, said he had to get back to take care of

his dogs. After a few minutes, the doctor convinced him now was the time to check it out.

The biopsy was done and sent to the pathologist. Clyde said he'd be back in three days for an appointment to find out the results of the biopsy.

Clyde didn't show up. They tried his phone but it had been disconnected. They sent him a letter urging him to come in and find out the results of the biopsy. He didn't come.

After a month they typed up a letter telling the patient that the biopsy was positive, that he had a malignancy and he should come in and talk about the next step, probably a radical prostatectomy. Time was a critical factor. They said the cancer had been caught quickly enough that it could probably be cured since it most likely hadn't spread outside the prostate.

Six months later the urologist realized that the man had not contacted them. The registered letter return receipt had come back from another state, so they knew the man had received the letter. He had been informed that he had prostate cancer.

He simply refused to face the reality that he had cancer and had to do something about it.

Arthur Z., 61, had a mild case of BPH. He got up once a night to urinate, had a small hesitancy problem and now and then felt like he couldn't empty out completely. He made it clear the first visit that he knew about the TURP and the open surgeries and didn't want any of them.

This was before the balloon dilation treatment. He wanted to try everything else. They started with Zinc and vitamins, which had a good effect for a while, whether a placebo effect or not he never could tell. Then that quit working and he wanted to test the bovine prostate regimen, which the urologist prescribed.

The bovine pills didn't seem to work so Arthur went back to the doctor. This time they tried bio-feedback training, but that didn't help him. Next they tried Alpha-One medication which didn't work either.

They went through most of the over-the-counter type pills and treatments, but every step of the way the urologist checked Arthur's kidney function to be sure there was no damage.

At last report Arthur was still trying new cures for his BPH, but his urologist was monitoring him. Arthur shrugged and grinned. "When it gets bad enough, I'll come in and we'll have the surgery. But not yet."

George C., 58, is president of his own firm and must do a lot of business entertaining. He has a moderate case of BPH but simply can't stop drinking any fluids after four in the afternoon. His clients wouldn't understand.

After several sessions with his urologist, they decided to try the balloon dilation treatment. George was told it could be done in the urologist's office, that it was a simple procedure, and if it worked on him, he should have no problem with the former BPH symptoms for up to three years.

During the interview before the operation, George agreed that if this didn't work, he'd come back for a TURP. He was at a point in his business that it was vital that he spend two to four nights a week with business prospects, eating, drinking and showing them a good time.

They scheduled the dilation and it went off well and without any complications. Three days later, George called the urologist and offered to buy him a drink that night. He felt like he was thirty again and he had no more BPH symptoms.

A year after his dilation, George sold his business for twelve million dollars and is now looking for another business challenge.

12

Answers to Some Questions You May Have

OKAY, SO I GET UP ONCE A NIGHT AND HESITATE A LITTLE WHEN I START TO URINATE. DOES THAT MEAN I MIGHT HAVE THIS BPH?

You're smart enough to know that those two symptoms might mean that you're developing some blockage in your urinary tract. Why take chances? If you haven't been having an annual physical with a regular digital prostate check, you definitely should go see your doctor. Take off a couple of hours and see the man, it could be a quick way to save your life.

YOU SAID MOST CANCER OF THE PROSTATE GIVES NO CLUES THAT IT'S THERE FOR A LONG TIME. IF I HAVE THIS BPH, ISN'T THAT A LEAD IN TO CANCER AS WELL?

No, no, a thousand times no. BPH has no relation to

cancer. Cancer of the prostate can originate in the same prostate, but there is no tie between the two. If you have BPH and you want more checks that it isn't cancerous, take a PSA blood test and get a transrectal ultrasound test.

HOW LONG CAN I HAVE BPH WITHOUT IT GETTING TO THE SURGERY STAGE?

Urologists say that a slow developing BPH could be tracked for ten to twelve years, perhaps more, before surgery would be needed. It depends on the patient's ability to "cope" with the symptoms which means how he adjusts his lifestyle to the symptoms. For example, can he give up drinking six cans of beer every night? Can he stop drinking caffeine beverages? Can he accept the idea that he needs to get up twice a night, and still stay happy? As long as there is no damage to the kidneys, the length of BPH development is strictly up to the attitude, stamina and psychological makeup of the patient.

WHAT WERE THOSE SYMPTOMS OF BPH AGAIN?

The usual symptoms for BPH include:

- Slowing of the stream of the urine's force.
- Hesitation to begin urinating.
- Inability to shut off urine. Involuntary dribbling after you try to stop it.
- A feeling that you have not emptied your bladder.
- Frequent urination during the day.
- Nocturia . . . frequent wakings during the night to urinate.
- A tightness and the inability to urinate at all.
- Nausea, dizziness, sleepiness if your kidneys have been damaged by urine retention.

I HATE GOING TO A DOCTOR. IF I HAVE TO GO

SEE A SPECIALIST, THIS UROLOGIST, WHAT DO I ASK HIM?

You don't have to worry, the urologist will be the one asking most of the questions. He has a long list. As he asks his questions a lot of yours will be answered. If they aren't, here are some points you might want to double check with him so you understand what's happening and what you can expect in the future.

1. What is this condition I have and what is it called?
2. Do I get some pills for it, or some other treatment, or will it clear up quickly by itself?
3. Are you going to give me any tests, and if so what kind? After that will I need checkups?
4. Do I have to have surgery? Is there another way to take care of my condition? If not, what are the risks of this surgery?
5. If I don't agree to any treatment or surgery, what can happen to me?
6. If I need surgery will it be in a hospital, in your office or as an outpatient?
7. If it's in a hospital, how long do I have to stay there?
8. When can I get back to work after the surgery?
9. How long after the surgery is it before I can have intercourse again?
10. Will this operation make me impotent? I hear all prostate stuff makes a guy sterile and unable to get an erection. Is that true?
11. A friend of mine had one of these and he says he ejaculates backwards. What does he mean?

SAY I DO HAVE THIS BPH THING. ARE THERE ANY DRUGS OR FOODS THAT I CAN'T TAKE OR USE ANY MORE?

Yes, there are several. Your doctor will be able to tell you exactly which ones might affect you. Here are some items that generally are not good for prostate patients:

Alcohol, anabolic steroids, nose sprays, heart and hypertension and ulcer medications, antidepressants, some cough medicines, tranquilizers and antihistamines.

Your doctor will be sure to advise you against the use of any of these depending on your individual situation.

I'M NOT MADE OUT OF MONEY. HOW MUCH DO THESE OPERATIONS COST? HOW MUCH IS A TURP AND HOW MUCH FOR A BALLOON DILATION?

Prices vary all over the country and from doctor to doctor within one city. A general price as quoted by one doctor in Minnesota was this: A balloon dilation for BPH costs about $3,600. A TURP closed operation with a two day hospital stay would cost about $12,000. Three times as much. However, remember that the balloon dilation is still in the experimental stage and the "feeling better" results may last only a few months and up to three years at the most. The TURP is done hundreds of thousands of times a year and usually is good for at least ten years.

HEY, IF THIS NEW DRUG HYTRIN IS SO GOOD, WON'T THAT JUST PUT AN END TO MOST OF THE TURP SURGERY? I MEAN, IF I CAN TAKE HYTRIN AND HAVE THE PROSTATE SHRINK AND MY BPH SYMPTOMS GO AWAY, I WON'T NEED SURGERY . . . WOW!

It would be great if true. But the fact is by mid 1993 Hytrin was in the very early stages of being used for BPH problems. For some it worked, for some it didn't. For some there were really bad side effects. It is no cure all. Just how well it's going to work won't be known for three or four years. By then there will be some testing and papers and reports and your urologist will know better how and when to use Hytrin and the other new one, Proscar. Proscar is in the last stages of the approval chain by the FDA and entered the market in 1993.

THIS TURP OPERATION. ARE THERE REALLY FIVE PERCENT OF THE PATIENTS WHO ARE IMPOTENT AFTER THE SURGERY?

The figure is between five and six percent, but remember, we're talking about men who average 67 years of age at the time of the operation. The statistic may be unreliable. A lot of men 67 may not be sure if they were impotent before the operation or not. And many might claim they could get an erection before the operation when they really couldn't. The subject is extremely sensitive and subjective.

I DON'T KNOW A UROLOGIST. HOW CAN I FIND ONE?

Your family doctor probably can recommend a urologist to you who he knows and has worked with before. This is the best way. If you're a member of an HMO, you will be assigned to an in-house urologist.

You might want to call the local medical society. Usually such groups will have a referral service and give you the names of three urologists in your immediate area.

Check your local library for a state medical directory of all state licensed physicians. Most are listed by specialty, such as urologists, and by city.

American Board of Certified Specialists is another directory you can find in your library. Here urologists are listed by states and communities. If the library doesn't have that one try for the American Medical Association directory.

WHAT ABOUT HELP AGENCIES FOR CANCER PATIENTS?

One of the best is the American Cancer Society. Its address is: American Cancer Society, National Headquarters, 4 West 35th Street, New York, NY 10001. The phone number is (212) 736-3030.

This national group funds its own research, supports research by other groups and has a number of patient support programs. Among them is the "I Can Cope" operation for patients and families. Its "CanSurmount" program is a patient-to-patient support service.

There are many local American Cancer Society groups that can help cancer patients. One of these programs is called "Road to Recovery" and helps with transportation. Some offer help with home care and financial aid.

Your local phone directory probably has a listing for the American Cancer Society. Give them a call for help with printed materials and what services they offer in your area.

The National Cancer Institute conducts research on cancer and supports other research facilities. They have an active reference and informational service for cancer patients and their families. They call it the CIS, Cancer Information Service, and it has a toll-free number:

(800) 4-CANCER . . . in U.S. and Puerto Rico.
(808) 524-1234 in Oahu, Hawaii.

A call to the cancer information number will tie in to the regional office of the NCI that serves your area. The person on the end of the line is trained to help you by providing answers to cancer related questions you might have. They also can tell you about local agencies and services to help you. On request they can tell you where the nearest medical library is to your home.

In some areas they will tell you about the closest Comprehensive Cancer Center and give you information about any experimental programs for prostate cancer then being given.

For more information from this group, including printed material on cancer of the prostate, contact them at: National Cancer Institute NCI, National Institutes of Health, Building 31, Room 1018A, Bethesda, MD 20014.

The Canadian Cancer Society is located at 130 Bloor Street West, Suite 1001, Toronto, Ontario, Canada M58-2V7. Their phone number is (416) 961-7223.

This society offers many programs similar to those of the American group. They have divisions in each of the provinces. Local phone directories should list the nearest office. If not, information operators can help you.

A Listing of Some Other Groups That May Be Able to Help You:

Information on Impotence, Incontinence, Sexuality.
The Simon Foundation
Box 835 Z
Wilmette, IL 60091
(800) 237-4666

The Simon Foundation offers a newsletter and several publications in the field of incontinence. It serves as a referral operation to individuals and has an informational service.

Impotence Institute International and Impotence Institute of America.
119 South Ruth Street

Maryville, TN 37801-5746
(615) 983-6064

The home of Impotents Anonymous, IA, for men, and I-ANON for the partners of impotent men.

This group was started in 1983 to educate and inform the public about the causes and treatment of impotence. It conducts and sponsors programs to carry out these ideals. They have a newsletter, and a videotape called, "Impotence, Help and Hope," that can be borrowed.

Their meetings are patterned after AA principles, and there are chapters across the country. The chapters use laymen as coordinators and have urologists as advisors and consultants at the meetings. For information send a self-addressed and stamped envelope to the address above.

ROMP (Recovery of Male Potency)
Grace Hospital
18700 Mayers Road
Detroit, MI 48235
(800) 835-7667

This hospital based group has chapters around the country and serves as a referral and information service. They also offer emotional support. Phoning the above number will put you in touch with a nurse. That person will refer you to a local source near you for help. There is a newsletter and other printed material available.

SIECUS (Sex Information and Education Council of the United States.)
80 Fifth Avenue
New York, NY 10011.

This organization furnishes information about periodicals, books and other groups involved with sexuality and sexual dysfunction. To get a list of sources in this field entitled: "Sexuality and Disability: A Bibliography of Resources Available for Purchase," send a stamped, self addressed #10 envelope and $1 to the address above.

AMERICAN ASSOCIATION OF SEX EDUCATORS, COUNSELORS AND THERAPISTS.
11 Dupont Circle N.W. Suite 220
Washington, DC 20036
(202) 462-1171

A certification group that approves sex counselor-therapists and can provide a list of these professionals in your area. Phone or write them for the information.

Other Health Groups:

* Food and Drug Administration
  Office of Consumer Communications
  Room 15B32 Parklawn Building
  5600 Fishers Lane
  Rockville, MD 20857

* Nutrition Foundation
  Suite 300
  888 Seventeenth St. N.W.
  Washington, D.C. 20006

* Mental Health Association
  1800 North Kent Street
  Arlington, VA 22209

* Office Of Health Information
  Office of the Surgeon General
  Department of Health, Education and Welfare
  Room 721BHHH
  200 Independence Ave. S.W.
  Washington, DC 20007

Recently a National Prostate Cancer week has been started. It's an awareness move that is good. Cancer research is stuck at about one percent for Prostate Cancer. That's not true at a new Foundation in California, named after and begun by a prostate cancer victim. The foundation was begun before Robert Mathews died of cancer. It is dedicated 100% to the research and cure of prostate cancer. For more information, write or call:

* Robert J. Mathews Foundation
  3435 American River Drive
  Sacramento, CA 95864
  (916) 972-7055

Makers of Sexual Prostheses and Other Devices:

For information about products in the sexual prostheses field, write to these manufacturers. Most will send patients information on their devices, and may know of surgeons in your area qualified to implant them.

- Dacomed Corporation
  1701 East 79th Street
  Minneapolis, MN 55425

- Impotence Information Center
  American Medical Systems
  PO Box 9
  Minneapolis, MN 5546

- Surgitek/Medical Engineering Corporation
  3037 Mount Pleasant Street
  Racine, WI 53404

- Osborn Medical Systems
  PO Box 1478
  Augusta, GA 30903

- Mentor Corporation
  600 Pine Avenue
  Goleta, CA 93117
- Response/KSI. Inc.
  889 South Matlack St.
  West Chester, PA 19382

13

Prostate Cancer Support Groups

Drug addicts do it, alcoholics do it, over eaters do it, and now all around the country there are springing up Prostate Cancer Support Groups. Good.

These groups serve men who have had prostate cancer, have had operations for it, are waiting for operations, or are waiting to see how tests come out.

Most of these groups are run by laymen or women, who get groups of concerned people together to network, to talk about mutual problems, talk about treatments and methods and simply how to cope with cancer of the prostate.

Some of them invite others with cancer beside prostate.

We know of two physicians who lead such groups. One is Dr. Roy E. Berger, MD from Smithtown, New York. The other is Dr. Israel Barken in San Diego.

Dr. Barken explained how his group got started. He had heard about other groups around the country and decided it was time for him to get one going in San Diego.

He photo copied some flyers and put them in the city libraries, handed them out to his patients and did a little spreading of the word.

On the day of the meeting fifteen men showed up. He had the first meeting on the Saturday after Good Friday. He said this might have some special significance.

To start off that first meeting Dr. Barken told the men to take out their calenders and mark the Saturday after Good Friday ten years from that day. They would have a reunion that day in the year two thousand. All of the men in the room were between 65 and 80 years old.

Everyone got excited, they jumped out of their seats and said "I'll be there. I promise that I'll be there." They all made the promise that they would meet there in ten years on the day after Good Friday.

To get the meeting going, the men stood one at a time and told the others what cancer he had and the treatment and how he felt at that time.

They watched a video by Dr. Bernard Siegel, "Love, Miracles and Medicine" and talked about it. Then they decided that they would meet every other month instead of every three months.

During the second meeting they all introduced themselves again and told what cancer they had so everyone could get better acquainted. At this session the group decided to make a list of subjects and problems that they would talk about in the next few meetings.

One of the men volunteered to help get out the mailing

notices for every meeting and keep track of the lists and do the work to keep the group going.

About half of the men there were patients of Dr. Barken and the other half were not. They decided to talk about specific problems that the prostate cancer caused them such as sexual functioning and incontinence.

This led to the idea that they should define the goal of the group. Just what was its purpose and what did they want to accomplish? One of the goals they established was to educate the public about prostate cancer and how to detect it.

The group decided to invite the men's wives to the meetings since they were affected by the disease. Someone suggested that they have a list of phone numbers that a cancer patient could call to talk with other patients when it came time for him to decide which kind of treatment he wanted.

Dr. Barken said the meetings so far had been great successes. The men stayed around in the hallway after the meeting talking to each other and exchanging information and experiences. One interesting element was that the men brought clippings from newspapers and magazines about prostate cancer treatments and cures to see what Dr. Barken thought of them.

The group decided to form a political action committee so they could send letters to their government officials about various problems the cancer patient had dealing with Medicare. For example they said Medicare won't pay for rectal ultrasound, an often used cancer test.

Dr. Barken said the first two meetings proved to be highly beneficial to the participants. The idea of sharing problems and solutions and ways of working around misfortunes had a strongly positive effect on the members.

He said the meetings were definitely not crying sessions. The men who attended came away with a good mental attitude. Dr. Barken said the group agreed to have speakers at some of the meetings, and at others share and talk and network and do some good mental therapy.

Now, after three years of these monthly meetings, Dr. Barken says they have about 300 members in the group and more than 100 come to each meeting. They are networking, helping each other, and learning more about their problems and the disease and what they can do to cope with the various associated problems.

Dr. Barken says that men with all kinds of prostate conditions come to the support group. Some have had the TURP treatment, others have had laser surgery or cryosurgery. Some have had radiation, and some have no major prostate troubles yet, but come to help or to learn more about prostate troubles. Some of those who come are due for prostate surgery soon.

He said that each new member has two "big brothers" assigned to him to help him, to be available for phone call advice, shoulder crying, or anything else the new member needs.

His group sponsors many activities including an annual holiday meeting in December. They went to see the motion picture *The Doctor,* about a physician who treated patients coldly, then got cancer himself and found out what it was like to be a patient. After the movie, they went to a restaurant and ate and talked about the movie and their own doctor-patient relationship. Dr. Barken said he plans to continue the group indefinitely.

Is There Such a Support Group Near You?

There very well may be. A newsletter called CANCER COMMUNICATION, now in its sixth year and published out of Grand Rapids, Michigan by a nonprofit corporation, recently printed a list of such groups around the country.

Lloyd Ney is the editor of the newsletter which is produced by Patient Advocates For Advanced Cancer Treatments, or PAACT. The editor says that PAACT's job is ". . . to educate the patient about the latest available information on the diagnosis and treatment of prostate cancer, without financial obligation . . ."

The newsletter covers a variety of new treatments, reports about conferences on cancer, letters to the editor about treatments that went wrong and more that went right. It's an interesting publication. The address is:

PATIENT ADVOCATES FOR ADVANCED
CANCER TREATMENTS (PAACT)
CANCER COMMUNICATIONS
PO BOX 1656
GRAND RAPIDS, MI 49504
Phone: (616) 453-1477

Self-Help Groups by States

A caution: moderators or administrators of the groups listed here may change from time to time. This list was up to date as we went to press in early 1993. If the phone number listed has changed for the person you need to contact in the city nearest you, please phone the

PAACT Michigan office number, (616) 453-1477, for current number in your area for the support group moderator.

If there is no group near you, you may want to call one of the other moderators in another city for advice how you can get a group going in your town through your urologist or a hospital or clinic.

ALABAMA

Wayne Martin, 25 Orchard Dr., Fairhope, AL 36532. (205) 928-3975

CALIFORNIA

Frank Bolle, PO Box 1525, Aptos, CA 95001. (408) 662-2437.

Norman Gollin, 9048 Wonderland Park Ave., Los Angeles, CA 90046. (213) 656-2398.

Bernard Safyan, 6667 Maryland Dr., Los Angeles, CA 90067. (213) 653-1401.

Thomas Van Straaten, 2326 Century Hill, Los Angeles, CA 90067. (213) 552-9830.

Michele Bonant, 12629 Riverside Dr., North Hollywood, CA 91607. (818) 753-2483.

Harry Reich, 6733 Colton Blvd., Oakland, CA 94611. (415) 339-9848.

Dr. James DeFranco, PO Box 1631, Palm Desert, CA 92261. (619) 568-4909.

Jack Marlin, 333 Merito Place, Palm Springs, CA 92262. (619) 325-5236.

Clarence Rath, 6442 Moss Lane, Paradise, CA 95969. (916) 877-8017.

Dee Israelson, 441 Wyndgate Rd., Sacramento, CA 96864. (916) 484-7075.
Dr. Israel Barken, 6600 Alvarado Road, San Diego, CA 92120. (619) 287-8866.
Marilyn Leve, PO Box 5234, San Pedro, CA 90733. (213) 831-5708.
Arthur De Manty, 2150 Cherry St., Sanger, CA 93657. (209) 875-5147.
Henry Wilder, 417 Monarch Bay, South Laguna, CA 92677. (714) 499-3945.
Francis Keryk, 1575 Benton St., Sunnyvale, CA 94087. (408) 243-9477.
Sharon McGowan, 350 N. Wiget Lane, S-10, Walnut Creek, CA 94598. (415) 933-0107.
Gilbert Draper, 9 Orchard Hill Road, Woodside, CA 94062. (415) 851-7574.

COLORADO

Harlow Sammons, 1336 Cherry, Denver, CO 80220. (303) 321-6273.

CONNECTICUT

Joann Gober, Box 63, Cromwell, CT 06416. (401) 364-3607.

DISTRICT OF COLUMBIA

John A. Baker, Sr., 3610 Idaho Ave. NW, Washington, DC 20016. (202) 966-3605.

FLORIDA

Otto J. Glasser, 4472 Highland Park, Sarasota, FL 34235. (813) 378-5065.

Zoltan George Horvath, 250 Kidd St., Ft. Walton Beach, FL 32548. (904) 664-5712.
Robert Windholz, 309 Springdale Drive, Bradenton, FL 34210. (813) 758-4195.
Leonard J. Smith, 451 Ives Dairy Road, Miami, FL 33179. (305) 654-4460.
Emmett Meyers, Rt. #10, 3225 110th Place, Vero Beach, FL 32963. (407) 589-8060.

ILLINOIS

Rev. Jack Pement, 216 Kenilworth Ave., Glen Ellyn, IL 60137. (708) 858-0366.
Albert Von Entress, 1544 Clyde Drive, Naperville, IL 60565. (708) 717-5554.

INDIANA

Dr. Bernard Vodnoy, 1430 E. Clayton Drive, South Bend, IN 46614. (219) 291-8773.

MARYLAND

Peter Weaver, 2 Wisconsin Circle, S 700, Chevy Chase, MD 20815. (301) 229-8730.

MAINE

Charles N. Green, RFD 5, Box 2477, Cundy's Harbor, Brunswick, ME 04011. (207) 729-6750.

MICHIGAN

Gary Albrecht, 200 Riverfront Park, 5A, Detroit, MI 48226. (no phone listed)
David Rogers, 37588 Windwood, Farmington Hills, MI 48024. (no phone listed)

Edwin T. McHenry, 340 N. Eagle St., Marshall, MI 49068. (616) 781-8622.
James Barber, 44599 Claire Blvd., Plymouth, MI 48170. (313) 453-9212.
A. W. "Bud" Irish, 705 Wilson, Saginaw, MI 48603. (517) 792-2157.
Wilbur Bernardi, 1481 E. Chateau Vert., Ypsilanti, MI 48197. (313) 434-6742.

MINNESOTA

Arnold A. Weiss, 5109 Meadow Ridge, Minneapolis, MN 55439. (612) 941-6955.
James Haddad, 910 Rice Creek Terrace, Fridley, MN 55432. (612) 571-9214.

MISSOURI

Alan E. Blum, 2217 Divot Drive, St. Louis, MO 63131. (314) 997-5013.

MISSISSIPPI

Langdon Herndon, PO Box 366, Gautier, MS 39553. (601) 497-3138.

NORTH CAROLINA

Arnold L. Aronson, 4401 W. Rowan St., Raleigh, NC 27609. (919) 787-4819.

NEW JERSEY

Robert L. Steiner, 406 Rosedale Rd., Princeton, NJ 08540. (609) 924-7184.

NEW YORK

John P. Pavacic, 114 Washington Ave., Patchogue, NY 11772. (516) 475-5772.
Dr. Roy Berger, 267C E. Main St., Smithtown, NY 11787. (516) 360-1266.
Averill Crane, 31 Oak Street, Smithtown, NY 11787. (516) 265-4660.
Mort Gimbel, 1776 Harvard Ave., Merrick, NY 11566. (516) 379-0853.
Julian Linker, 636 Diane Place, North Woodmere, NY 11581. (516) 791-2776.
Dr. Kurt Wasserman, 382 Central Park West, #19H, New York City, NY 10025. (212) 932-1976.

OHIO

James W. Broad, 333 Duane Street, Clyde, OH 43410. (419) 547-7942.
Lawrence W. Miller, 421 Roshon Drive, Medina, OH 44256. (216) 725-7387.
Robert Kanter, 7434 Aracoma Drive, Cincinnati, OH 45237. (513) 531-3711.

OREGON

James Snow, 3901 SW Bridlemile Court, Portland, OR 97221. (503) 227-3901.
Jack Plemmons, 11865 SW Wilkens Lane, Beaverton, OR 97005. (503) 524-8722.

PENNSYLVANIA

Craig Waldner, 820 Old Washington Rd., McMurray, PA 15317. (412) 941-7331.
James Conway, RD #2, Irish Road, Edinboro, PA 16412. (814) 734-4370.

Dr. Suresht P. Amina, 2000 Green Street, Farrell, PA 16121. (412) 981-3443.

SOUTH CAROLINA

Donald Cobble, 916 Misty Harbor Rd., Chapin, SC 29036. (803) 345-3484.

TENNESSEE

Harry Daugherty, Jr., PO Box 6306, Chattanooga, TN 37401. (615) 265-2574.

TEXAS

Peter A. A. Raines, 2807 Arroyo Court N., College Station, TX 77845. (409) 764-7581.
Dr. David Capper, 700 W. Rosedale, Fort Worth, TX 76104. (817) 335-2161.
Martin Davidson, 3636 Haynie Ave., Dallas, TX 75205. (214) 361-5638.

VIRGINIA

Arthur Weinfield, 3918 Lake Blvd., Annandale, VA 22003. (703) 280-9820.
Dr. Rene B. Alvir, 611 S. Carlin Springs Rd., Arlington, VA 22204. (708) 671-7717.
Charles Pitchford, 220 Granby Park, Norfolk, VA 23505. (804) 917-2560.

WASHINGTON

Dr. Richard Swanson, 1402 W. Lake Sammamish Rd., SE, Belleview, WA 98008. (206) 746-3999.
John Farrell, 27833 10th Ave. S., Feceral Way, WA 98003. (206) 839-4787.

WISCONSIN

Evan "Red" Vogds, 346 Ellis, Fond-du-Lac, WI 54935. (414) 921-5808.

Dennis "Doc" Schultz, 366 Roosevelt, Fond-du-Lac, WI 54935. (414) 921-9432.

Warren Drumm, 319 S. 10th Ave., Wausau, WI 54401. (715) 848-6141.

John R. Moulton, 310 E. Sunset Ct., Madison, WI 53705. (608) 231-2757.

Glossary

(Note: All of these words may not be used in this book, but they may come up in talks with your urologist, doctor or nurse. This list will give you a ready reference as a layman in a medical world.)

abscess: An accumulation of pus that might result in swelling, fever, and pain.

accessory sex gland: A mass of glandular tissue that plays a secondary role in reproduction.

acid phosphatase: An enzyme made in the prostate gland.

acute: Reaching a crisis rapidly, quick, sudden. Having a short and relatively severe course.

acute bacterial prostatitis: See: Prostatitis.

adenoma: A benign tumor where cells form recognizable glandular structures.

alkaline phosphatase: An enzyme made by the liver, bone and other bodily structures.

ampulla: A small dilation in a canal or duct.

androgens: Bodily hormones that help the development and maintenance of the male sex characteristics. One of these is testosterone. The lack of sufficient androgens causes the prostate to shrink.

anesthetic: A substance that causes the loss of nerve responses in part or all of the body. A general anesthetic results in unconsciousness. A local anesthetic causes a small area to lose its sensitivity to pain. A spinal anesthetic is in the subarachnoid space around the spinal cord.

antihistamine: Any drug used to relieve symptoms of allergies and colds. They work by neutralizing the effects of histamine, one of the active substances in allergic reactions.

antihormones: Drugs used to block hormones that stimulate cancer growth.

anus: The exterior opening at the end of the digestive tract. Through it waste products are excreted.

artery: A blood vessel (hollow tube) that carries blood from the heart to bodily tissue.

aspiration: A method to remove fluids, gases, tissue or cells from a body cavity by the use of suction.

atrophy: The shrinking or wasting of tissues, organs, muscles or the entire body. A man's testes will atrophy leaving the scrotum intact if male hormones are withheld from him or if he is given female hormones.

artificial uninary sphincter: A special prosthesis designed to bring back urine control in an incontinent person by constricting the urethra.

bacteria: A broad class of unicellular microorganisms. Some live and feed off other living things. Many, but not all of them, cause diseases in man and animals.

bacterial prostatitis: An infection taking place in the prostate gland caused by bacteria.

bacteriuria: When the urine shows the presence of bacteria.

benign: Not malignant. Characteristic of a mild illness. Favorable for recovery.

benign prostatic hyperslasia (BPH): The growth and enlargement of the glandular tissue within the prostatic capsule. This growth usually pushes the lobes of the prostate against the urethra causing urination problems. This growth is not cancerous.

bilateral: Being made up of or having two related sides.

biopsy: The removal of tissue from a living patient so it can be studied to establish a precise diagnosis.

bladder: A sack to hold something. Here an elastic sac that serves to store urine before it is excreted from the body.

bladder neck: The opening in the bladder that meets the urethra through which urine flows.

bladder spasm : A sudden, involuntary contraction of the bladder muscles that produces pain and problems with urination.

*blood urea nitrogen (BUN):*A blood test used to measure proper kidney functioning.

blood acid phosphatase level: The relative amount of phosphatase in a patient's blood. It's an enzyme. An increase of this acid phosphatase in blood can indicate cancer of the prostate has spread to other areas.

blood cells: The cells, along with plasma make up human blood. They are manufactured in the bone marrow and may be white blood cells, red blood cells or platelets.

body imaging: Any technique that produces a picture of the body's interior such as X-rays, CAT scans, MIR and ultrasound.

boggy: Said of the prostate when it is swollen, spongy and soft.

bone scan: An image of the body's bones made by injecting the patient with a radioactive chemical that travels to the areas around the bones, highlighting any bone irregularity, injury or problem. Used to detect prostate cancer that has spread to bones.

bone survey: A series of X-rays of the complete skeletal system. Used in diagnosing and locating cancer that has spread.

BPH: See: Benign Prostatic Hyperplasia.

cancer: The uncontrolled growth of abnormal cells creating a cellular tumor. Such cells invade other cells and tissue and can spread throughout the body through the blood stream or lymphatic system.

capsule: The structure in which an item is enclosed, such as the prostate capsule.

cardiovascular: Dealing with the heart, the blood vessels and with circulation.

catheter: A hollow, flexible surgical tube for introducing or withdrawing liquids, wastes, or instruments in the body. Especially used through the urethra into the bladder to drain urine.

CAT scan: A technique using X-rays and computer technology to do an imaging of the body to provide a highly informational cross section picture.

chlamydia: A group of spherical-shaped nonbacterial organisms that can cause infection in the urethra.

chronic bacterial prostatitis: The bacterial infection of the prostate that continues over a long period of time.

coitus: Sexual intercourse.

coitus interruptus: The deliberate withdrawal of the penis during intercourse before ejaculation.

coitus prolongus: The deliberate holding off of ejaculation during intercourse.

compensated: A bladder that empties completely during normal urination.

congestion: A swelling due to increased blood in the body's vessels or tissue.

congestive prostatitis: A form of prostatitis that is not

due to infection but may be caused by stress, chronic vibration, sexual habits.

contraceptive: Any device, drug or behavior designed to prevent pregnancy.

contrast medium: A dye used in veins to highlight structures of the kidney and related tubes for visualization and X-rays and other imaging means.

cryosurgery: The use of a probe that releases ultra cold liquid nitrogen for surgery of the prostate for BPH and for cancer.

cystoscope: A lighted instrument that is passed into the urethra for examining the urethra and the bladder.

decompensated bladder: A bladder that can't totally empty during urination leaving residual urine in the bladder.

digital rectal examination: The examination of the prostate done by inserting a finger into the rectum and touching the two outer lobes of the prostate.

dribbling: (regarding urination) An involuntary stream or drops of urine at the conclusion of urination.

-ectomy: An ending to a word which means surgical removal. Combined with a part of the body such as: prostatectomy, tonsillectomy.

ejaculation: The act of emission of semen from the penis.

erectile dysfunction: The inability of the penis to achieve sufficient stiffness for vaginal penetration.

erection: The stiffening and enlargement of the penis when it becomes filled with blood during sexual arousal.

estrogens: A combining term for female sex hormones. Several have different functions but they are closely related and collectively they are called estrogen. Estrogen enables a woman to develop reproductive organs and secondary sex characteristics. Synthetic estrogens are sometimes used to shrink the male testes in cancer treatments.

excision: Removal of tissue or a part of the body surgically.

external radiation: Radiation from a machine outside the body aimed at a cancer within the body.

external urethral sphincter: A band of muscle fibers that are voluntarily constricted or relaxed to allow or restrict the flow of urine from the bladder out of the body through the penis.

fertile: Capable of conceiving and bearing children.

fiber optics: The type of optics that uses a flexible tube containing glass or plastic fibers that transmit and bend light and reflect a magnified image. Instruments using fiber optics can be inserted into the urethra and the urologist can see the inside of the tube and determine any blockage.

flow rate, urine: How quickly urine is voided from the bladder at the peak period of urination. If it's lower than the average, it may mean some urethral obstruction is present.

foreskin: A free fold of skin that covers or partly covers the head of the penis when it is flaccid. The foreskin is partly or entirely removed in circumcision.

frequency: In urology the need to urinate at short intervals.

genitals, genitalia: The reproductive organs of the male and female both internal and external.

genitourinary: The reproductive and urinary tract of a man, the specialty of the urologist along with the urinary tract of a woman.

gland: An organ that utilizes material from the blood and converts it into new compounds which then can be secreted internally or returned to the bloodstream.

glans: A roughly triangular structure on the male called the glans penis on the end of the penis. In the female the glans clitoridis is a small mass of tissue at the tip of the clitoris that can become erect.

gynecologist: A medical doctor who specializes in the reproductive system, diseases, and endocrinology of women.

gynecomastia: The unnatural development or enlargement of breasts in men sometimes the result of estrogen treatments.

hematuria: Blood in the urine.

hemospermia: Blood in the seminal fluid.

hesitancy: A slowness to start the urinary stream.

hormonal therapy: The treatment of cancer or other diseases or conditions through the use of hormones.

hormone: A compound from the endocrine glands that is circulated through the body in the bloodstream. Each has a specific nature and function.

hypertrophy: The excessive growth or development of an organ or part; exaggerated growth or complexity.

impotence: The inability of a man to achieve and sustain an erection sufficient for vaginal penetration.

incontinent: A person's inability to control the voiding of urine or feces.

infection: The invasion of microorganisms of some bodily part or section where they grow and produce toxins that injure the tissue.

infectious prostatitis inflammation: Prostatitis caused by an invasion of yeast, viruses, or bacteria in the prostate. Symptoms include redness, heat, swelling, and pain and are the result of some injury, irritation or infection.

intermittency: The inability to void completely and empty the bladder on one contraction of the bladder, resulting in a stopping and starting of the urinary flow.

internal radiation: Radiation treatment through the use of radioactive "seeds" with a life expectancy of 17 to 34 days that are implanted in a cancerous tumor such as one in the prostate.

intravenous pyelogram: X-ray pictures taken after the injection of dyes intravenously into the bloodstream. The X-ray pictures outline the parts of the urinary tract and help in diagnosis.

kidneys: Two small organs located on each side of the

spinal column. Through them the blood impurities are removed and dissolved to form urine.

laser: Stands for: Light Amplification by Stimulated Emission of Radiation. Laser beams are concentrated light and heat and can be used to cut much like a scalpel. More and more are now used in surgery internally where a scalpel can't reach.

lateral lobes: Of the prostate. They usually grow after a man reaches forty and often squeeze the urethra and cause the problem known as BPH.

lesion: A wound or injury. In cancer, a mass of cells that may be semisolid or solid, inflammatory, malignant or benign.

leydig cells: Cells in the testes that produce testosterone.

libido: Sexual desire, whether conscious or unconscious.

lobes of the prostate: Five lobes make up the prostate, two lateral, a middle, a posterior and the anterior. When the two lateral and the middle lobes enlarge they can produce BPH symptoms.

localized: With cancer cells, said to remain at the site of the original malignancy and not spreading.

lymph nodes: A whole network of small masses of lymphoid tissue throughout the body. They are a defense mechanism by removing bacteria and other toxins from surrounding tissue, and supplying lymphocytes to the blood.

MRI: Magnetic Resonance Imaging. Produces a cross sectional image of the body much like the CAT scan.

Can detect dead or degenerating cells, blockage of blood and cancer. Extremely expensive. One MRI machine costs around $3 million.

male hormones: The androgen hormones that make a man a man. Two of them: androsterone and testosterone.

malignant: Cancerous as in malignant tumor. Having the ability of invasion of other tissues and metastases (spreads) through the body.

masturbation: The stimulation of one's own or another's genital organs, other than in intercourse, for sexual gratification.

metabolism: The physical and chemical processes needed to maintain life and to produce changes in tissue. Some types break down large particles into smaller ones to provide energy to the body. Others convert small particles into larger ones for storing energy.

metastasis: The spread of cancerous cells and the resulting tumors to other parts of the body from the original source. This is usually done by either the bloodstream or the lymph system or both.

neoplasm: A tumor of new growth or abnormal growth. Also it can be swelling of tissue. This can be either malignant or benign.

nephritis: Chronic or acute inflammation of the kidneys.

nocturia: An urge to urinate so strong that it wakes you up at night from a sound sleep.

nodule: A small tumor or mass of tissue, usually malignant but not always.

nonbacterial prostatitis: Prostate inflammation but without any known bacterial cause.

nocturnal emission: A wet dream. The discharge of semen during sleep. A natural way to rid the body of excess fluid in the prostate. Can also result from erotic dreams.

nuclear scan: A test using radioactive trace compounds for diagnosis.

occult prostatic carcinoma: Cancer of the prostate that is not suspected but is found after prostate surgery for BPH. Usually a stage A cancer.

oncology: The treatment and study of neoplasms and cancerous tumors. An oncologist is a physician trained to treat these cancers.

orchiectomy: Surgery in which both or one testicle is removed. When done for cancer of the prostate, the scrotum is left in place.

orgasm: The ultimate release of the sexual act, often accompanied by strong muscular contractions, pleasurable sensations, and release of tensions. Ejaculation usually occurs for men. The male orgasm may take place without an erection.

palliative treatment: Medical care not aimed at curing the patient, but to make him feel better by relieving discomfort, pain or symptoms of a disease, condition or disorder.

palpation: A method where the physician uses hands, not instruments, to determine the size, texture, consistency and location of organ soreness, pain or growths.

PAP test: Prostate Acid Phosphatase test. A blood test given to check on the chance that a malignancy has spread out of the prostate into other parts of the body. An elevated reading here can indicate that movement of the cancer.

pathology: Deals with the physical results of disease in cells, organs and tissues that can be determined, evaluated and recorded through testing and microscopic examination.

peak urine flow: The maximum amount of urine flow that a patient can produce. Measured in milliliters per second.

penile prosthesis: Material inserted into the corpora cavernosa of the penis to make the organ rigid enough for vaginal penetration.

penis: The male sex organ used for urinary discharge and for sexual intercourse.

perineal prostatectomy: Surgery to remove all or part of the prostate gland. The incision is in the perineum.

perineum: That portion of the body between the scrotum and the anus.

pituitary gland: The endocrine gland situated at the base of the brain that produces hormones. These hormones regulate the secretions from other endocrine glands in the body.

potency: The ability of a male to achieve and maintain an erection and vaginal penetration.

prognosis: A doctor's best judgement of the probable outcome of a medical condition or disease.

prostate gland: A gland about the size of a walnut just below the bladder that surrounds the urethra. It makes most of the fluid that the spermatozoa travel in down the urethra and out the penis. The gland consists of connective tissue, muscle and glandular tissue. The glandular tissue makes the prostatic fluid.

prostatectomy: A surgical process that removes all or part of the prostate gland. Most performed is the TURP, or transurethral resection. Also done are the retropubic and suprapubic surgeries.

prostatic massage: A procedure where a digital rectal finger massages each of the lateral lobes to force secretions into the urethra and out of the body to relieve a congested prostate.

prostatitis: Inflammation of the prostate gland that can be acute, chronic or temporary. Usually caused by infection, irritation or congestion.

prostatostasis: A congested prostate gland with prostatic secretions often due to irregular, or infrequent ejaculations.

prosthesis: Any artificial device to replace a missing or malfunctioning part of the body.

PSA test: A blood test given to show the Prostate Specific Anigen level. A high level suggests that there is the presence of a cancerous growth in the prostate.

pubis: That area just above the external genitals.

pyuria: A condition when white blood cells, often pus cells, show up in the urine.

radiation: Energy that is emitted in the form of waves or particles such as X-rays, light, short radio or ultraviolet. Used in medicine for treatment and diagnosis.

radio-immuno assay: A method for measuring minute quantities of antigen or antibody, hormones and some drugs found in the body.

radiotherapy: The use of radiation in treatment of diseases.

rectal examination: For the prostate, the use of a finger in the rectum to feel the prostate gland testing for BPH and cancer.

rectum: The end portion and exterior opening of the large intestine.

renal scans: Produce two-dimensional picture from the gamma rays emitted by a radioactive isotope. Usually concentrated in a specific tissue of the body such as the kidney. They show blood flow to the kidney, and the function and any obstruction to kidney drainage.

refractory period: The time a man needs after ejaculation before he can achieve a second erection.

resection, transurethral: Removal of obstructing BPH prostate tissue with instruments inserted through the urethra.

resectoscope: A surgical instrument used in a transurethral resection of the prostate allowing the surgeon to see inside the urethra.

residual urine: Any urine left in the bladder after voiding. Normal residual amount is zero cc.

retention, urine: The inability to urinate when the bladder is full. Often caused by obstruction to the urethra due to BPH.

retrograde ejaculation: The flow of semen into the bladder instead of out the penis during ejaculation. Usually the result of a TURP operation where the bladder neck is damaged or removed, or the bladder neck is too weakened to close.

retropubic prostatectomy: Removal of some or all of the prostate gland due to BPH through an incision in the lower abdomen below the navel.

scan: A computerized display of an organ or part of the body shown by injecting radioactive substances into the patient. Helps diagnose and track tumors.

scrotum: A man's external pouch at his crotch that contains the testes and accessory organs.

secretions, prostatic: Fluid that is continuously produced from within the many glands of the prostate.

seminal fluid: Emitted by the penis during ejaculation. A thick, white fluid containing the spermatozoa. Contains fluids from the testes, the seminal vesicles, the prostate gland and the Cowper's gland.

seminal vesicles: A pair of small pouches behind the bladder that provides nutrient material for the sperm. It empties into the urethra at the time of ejaculation.

septic: A medical term meaning infection in the bloodstream.

sexual dysfunction: In the male, the inability to have an erection, to maintain it and penetrate the vagina, or not able to ejaculate, are all dysfunctions.

silent prostatism: Created when serious prostatic obstructions exist without showing any symptoms. Without treatment the condition can lead to serious kidney damage.

sitz bath: A hot water sit down bath that can have comforting effects for many types of rectal and urinary problems.

skinny needle prostatic aspiration: A very slender needle used to probe suspicious areas of the prostate, or other aspiration parts of the body, to retrieve biopsy samples.

sonogram: A computer printout that uses ultrasound waves to show the position, form and function of parts of the body. A sonogram can be printed out or recorded on a video tape for closer study.

sperm: The mature male germ cell which has a head and tail, which can fertilize the female ovum. Produced by the testes and contains the genetic input from the father given to the offspring.

sphincter, urinary: A ring-like muscle a man contracts when he shuts off his urine flow. Surrounds the urethra just beyond the prostate gland toward the penis.

staging: A medical term used to determine the extent of a patient's disease. In prostatic cancer to determine if the cancer is confined to the prostatic capsule.

sterile: The inability to produce offspring.

sterilization: An operation that makes a man unable to

produce offspring, such as removal of the testicles.

stilbestrol: A man-made female hormone sometimes given to men with prostatic cancer.

stones, bladder: The hard crystallization of urine in the bladder or from stones from the kidneys.

stricture: Medically the narrowing of a structure or passageway.

suprapubic prostatectomy: Surgical removal of all or part of the prostate gland by means of an incision below the navel and above the pubis in the lower abdomen.

testes, testicles: The two reproductive glands of the male situated in the scrotum. They produce sperm and androgens.

testosterone: The major male hormone for development of the male sex characteristics.

tissue: A group of similar cells united in a specific performance of a particular function.

trabeculation, bladder: The buildup of the bladder muscle due to obstruction to the slow flow of urine because of BPH.

transrectal: Going through the rectum, as a probe or a digital examination.

transurethral: Going through the urethra. Such as a catheter or instruments for a TURP surgery.

transurethral resection prostate: Also called TURP. The removal of all or part of the prostate by inserting an instrument through the urethra in the penis and cutting away the prostate tissue.

trigone, bladder: The highly sensitive portion of the bladder at the base of the sac which triggers the need to urinate.

true capsule prostate: The tough layer of tissue that surrounds the outside of the prostatic tissue.

true-cut biopsy needle: The most used hollow needle to remove a core of tissue from the prostate, or any part of the body, to see if it is cancerous or not.

tumor: The abnormal and excessive growth of tissues. Tumors can be either malignant or benign.

ultrasound: See sonogram.

uremia: The excess of nitrogen and urea in the blood. Leads to uremic poisoning. Can result in nausea, vomiting, dizziness, coma, convulsions and death.

urethra: The tube through which urine passes from the bladder to the outside through the penis. In men, seminal fluids as well flow through the urethra.

urine: Waste fluid that is all water but four percent, urine is excreted by the kidneys, sent to the bladder for storage and then expelled on demand through the urethra. The other four percent are dissolved substances from the body.

urine analysis: The chemical, physical and microscopic examination of the urine.

urine culture: The study of a urine sample at a determined temperature in a specific media to permit growth of microorganisms so they can be identified. This permits an exacting diagnosis of a urinary tract infection.

urologist: A physician specializing in the treatment of diseases of the urinary tract in males and females and the reproductive system in males.

vagina: The female genital canal leading from the uterus to the external bodily orifice.

vas deferens: Two tubes that propel and transport spermatozoa from the epididymis into the urethra.

vasectomy: The removal surgically of a section of both vas deferens which results in male sterility.

veins: Blood vessels that carry blood on its return trip from the capillaries back to the heart.

venereal disease: One of several diseases transmitted through sexual relations.

weak urinary stream: A male's urination flow that has less stream than normal force. A urologist measures this flow in milliliters per second.

workup: A complete medical picture of a patient from the combined results of examinations and tests, which help the physician to arrive at a diagnosis and treatment regimen.

X-ray: Any of several electromagnetic radiations of short wavelength, that penetrate muscle and bone and leave relative shadows. Useful in diagnostic medical work.

Index